AMERICA'S
MISUNDERSTOOD
WELFARE STATE

AMERICA'S MISUNDERSTOOD WELFARE STATE:

Persistent Myths, Enduring Realities

THEODORE R. MARMOR,
JERRY L. MASHAW,
AND
PHILIP L. HARVEY

BasicBooks
A Division of HarperCollins*Publishers*

Library of Congress Cataloging-in-Publication Data
Marmor, Theodore R.
      America's misunderstood welfare state: persistent
   myths, enduring realities / Theodore R. Marmor,
   Jerry L. Mashaw, and Philip L. Harvey.
         p. cm.
      Includes bibliographical references and index.
      ISBN 0-465-05969-4: $22.95
      1. United States—Social policy.   2. Public
   welfare—United States.   3. Social
   security—United States.   4. Medicare.   5. Welfare
   state.   I. Mashaw, Jerry L.   II. Harvey,
   Philip L.   III. Title.
   HN59.2.M374   1990   90-80240
   361.6'1'0973—dc20   CIP

To Elizabeth Auld

Contents

List of Figures

List of Tables

Preface

As the United States enters the 1990s, domestic social policy
seems likely, once again, to emerge as a major battleground.
While large budget deficits will continue to constrain federal
politics, there are unresolved social concerns that will be difficult to keep off the domestic agenda. The most pressing of these
will almost certainly be health care—its extraordinary cost, its
incomplete coverage, and its seeming imperviousness to reform. Homelessness, worries about the "underclass," and complex questions about the financing of Social Security will also
command attention. While the topics to be addressed seem
clear, what will be done about them is not, and it seems inevitable that the political legacy of the 1970s and 1980s will greatly
influence the working out of this domestic agenda.

The legacy includes an unflattering portrait of American social policy as a failed enterprise—unaffordable, unmanageable,
and undesirable. This portrayal, in our view, is both factually
questionable and interpretively misleading. It is not true that
American social programs were subject to uncontrolled growth
and unresponsive to straitened economic circumstances. It is
not the case that our social welfare budget is unaffordable, either in the sense that we are unwilling to pay for it or because

it is driving us to economic ruin. It is also demonstrably untrue that the Great Society initiatives of the 1960s exacerbated the conditions they were meant to address. Finally, it is simply wrongheaded to claim that the programs on which we spend most of our social welfare dollars—pensions and medical care—are unpopular, unneeded, or fraudulent.

Despite the fact that we spend considerable time defending American social welfare programs against criticism we believe is false, ours is not an argument for the status quo. Although we believe that the American welfare state has been unjustly maligned, we do not believe that it is free of serious troubles. Our reform ideas, however, are not based on a castigation of existing programs. Indeed, one of the features we find pernicious in American social policy debate is the assumption that reform proposals must be prefaced by trashing existing arrangements. Of course those who want to dismantle the welfare state will heap scorn on it. But it is both unnecessary and counterproductive for those who want to strengthen the welfare state to do the same.

We do not assume that the discarding of outworn shibboleths, by itself, will result in the implementation of better social policy. Nor will a better understanding of the commitments and successes of the American welfare state lead unerringly to a better tomorrow. Success in social welfare policy-making is never the simple result of analytical clarity. The complex federalism of American government and other features of our political life will continue to shape the course of our social policy and to limit possibilities for reform.

The twentieth century has brought dramatic changes to the organization of industrial society. More or less elaborate social welfare systems are now a universal and essential feature of a modern nation. The United States is no exception, but we have had more trouble than most countries in coming to terms with this development. Relentless negativism in our public debate about social policy adds unnecessary anxiety to necessary adjustment. It causes us to undervalue what we have accomplished and inhibits us from measured adaptations of our welfare state to changing circumstances. It is for these reasons that we believe an attempt to correct popular misconceptions of American social welfare policy is important.

ACKNOWLEDGMENTS

This book has extensive intellectual and institutional roots. Yale's Institution for Social and Policy Studies provided a congenial setting in the mid-1980s for a faculty seminar on Social Security that greatly strengthened our collaborative resolve. We are particularly grateful to Richard Nelson, then the director of ISPS, for nurturing this and other welfare state studies. Along the way, others contributed financial assistance to projects which in turn helped lead to this book. We acknowledged in an earlier book the help of the Ford Foundation and the philanthropic team of Alan Pifer and Forrest Chisman, but one thing did lead to another, and we want to note that earlier assistance.

The institution that made the greatest difference to this book is the Russell Sage Foundation. A fellowship in 1987–88 permitted one of us a year's leave to write the first draft at the foundation's special retreat in the middle of Manhattan. Beyond that was a continuing seminar on welfare state issues that gave all of us a forum in which to present the book's arguments and ample occasion for discussion with colleagues sharing similar interests. We want to thank the officers of Russell Sage, particularly Eric Wanner and Peter DiJanosi, both for supporting the writing of this book and for sustaining a setting so congenial to the task. We also acknowledge the special assistance we received from the Canadian Institute for Advanced Research. A fellowship to Marmor that began in 1988 gave our enterprise considerable support in research time and assistance. Finally, we are very grateful to the Rockefeller Foundation for that precious form of assistance, the small but unrestricted grant at the early stages of a difficult project.

More people read and commented on our drafts than is easy to remember, let alone acknowledge: Deborah Chassman, Fay Cook, Sandy Jencks, Rudolf Klein, Larry Mead, Ed Pauly, Jonathon Rieder, Aaron Wildavsky, Robert Morris, Michael Wolfson, Fraser Mustard, Robert Myers, Jill Quadagno, Sharon Russell, Laura Marmor, and Vee Burke. Others have read chapters or heard versions presented in various workshops and seminars. They may be surprised with the final result, but we remain indebted to them for taking the time to help us. Paul Pierson, Anne MacClintock, Jan Marmor, and Deborah Stone went over the last draft with special care and we are especially grateful to them. We also thank Susan Rose-Ackerman, Robert Ellickson, and Bruce Ackerman, Yale colleagues who reviewed the entire manuscript in penultimate form. Liz McGrath's research assistance was of great value during the writing of the first draft as was Andrew Tully's careful preparation of the final figures. Later on, the workshop audiences that responded to our presentations—at the Universities of Indiana, Minnesota, Toronto, and Wisconsin, as well as the London School of Economics—reinforced our urge to finish through support or criticism. Our editor at Basic Books, Martin Kessler, supplied the right mix of inducement, comment, and puzzlement to keep the project going. We are grateful to him, as are many writers about public life, for sustaining at Basic Books a powerful interest in modern governance.

One person, however, requires a very special acknowledgment. Elizabeth (Biz) Auld made contributions to this book so substantial that it would embarrass us, and perhaps her, to describe them in detail. Researcher and editor, typist and faxer,

organizer and retriever, enforcer of deadlines and expediter
of drafts, she made sure this book, so long in the making, got
finished. The advantages of joint authorship are considerable,
especially with a topic as wide-ranging as the American welfare state. But the costs of coordinating are considerable as
well and, in dedicating this book to her, we acknowledge as
forcefully as we can how grateful all three of us are for a level
of loyalty, conscientiousness, and competence no one has the
right to expect.

THEODORE R. MARMOR
JERRY L. MASHAW
PHILIP L. HARVEY
New Haven
June, 1990

1

Social Welfare Policy under Siege

This book has a simple message: America's social welfare efforts are taking a bum rap.[1] Our social programs, however successful in practice, are now typically portrayed as failures, almost never as sources of pride. Persistent pessimism, usually the preserve of antigovernment ideologues, has characterized the general tone of social welfare policy discussion over the past two decades, with elite criticism both stimulating and reflecting popular dismay. A 1976 Harris poll, for example, found that only 13 percent of those surveyed expressed "great confidence" in the Congress and the executive branch, down nearly 30 percent from a decade earlier.[2] During the 1970s, mocking President Lyndon Johnson's "Great Society" programs was a favorite political sport—inviting targets, perhaps, because of Johnson's overblown rhetoric. Even former supporters of activist government efforts to combat social ills publicly announced their dismay at "the failure of so many of the government programs they once cherished," and their frustration that "the social problems that [liberal programs of the 1960s] were supposed to solve remain."[3] What disillusioned liberals regretted, longtime critics of social policy proclaimed with enthusiasm: the Great Society had failed.[4] In the 1980s, the war on Washington continued, led during two presidential terms by Ronald Reagan.

For much of the period since the early 1970s, therefore, Americans have heard a chorus of complaints about their government, with especially harsh words for the transfer programs that account for over 40 percent of federal spending. The administration of George Bush has promised to be "kinder and gentler," but its major social policy preoccupation has been a "war" on drugs that, given the Panama invasion of December 1989, it seems to have meant quite literally. There is now an almost paradoxical disjunction between the rhetoric and the reality of the American welfare state.

Yet this new consensus on social welfare policy hides more than it reveals. The reality of government efforts generally, and of social programs in particular, is not one of unmitigated failure. And, although many Americans share the critical views of elite commentators in the abstract, their opinions concerning the specific major programs of the American welfare state are overwhelmingly favorable (see discussion in chapter 2). The vision of social welfare policy generated during these two decades thus has often been misleading and misdirected, indeed, riddled with myths.

We have been puzzled about why the social policy debate should have taken on such a distorted cast. There is, to be sure, much myth-making in the whole of American public life. Social facts are elusive, and economic information hardly interprets itself. We should expect stories, parables, and myths to be partial guides where the social, economic, and political reality is disputable. But the necessity of story making does not in itself require such dark tales, such dismal accounts of American social welfare policy. Why do we find so many tales of failure and disappointment rather than stories that mix accomplishment, even transcendence, with the undeniable difficulties?[5]

IDEOLOGY MATTERS

How are we to explain contemporary concern expressed by politicians, social commentators, and even the proverbial person in the street about "the welfare mess," and the "failures of the Great Society?" Why do economists, investment bankers, political scientists, newspaper editors—even an occasional safe, foolish, or retired politician—bemoan the "sacred cow" status of Social Security pensions, or talk in apocalyptic tones about the "coming crash" or the "intergenerational time bomb" created by the structure or financing of our social insurance programs? Could all this doom and gloom really be warranted? If not, why is the dismay so prevalent?

There are many plausible answers to this question. One is that Americans are perfectionist and impatient. We find fault with everything on the way to reforming or improving it.[6] We are little disposed to backward-looking self-congratulation. Indeed, finding fault and proposing reform are institutionalized in a reformist press and in an accusatory, reform-minded electoral politics. Given these propensities, social welfare programs are likely to get more than their fair share of criticism. As even critics acknowledge, the broadest goal of social welfare policy is heroic—to secure all of us from want. The very elusiveness of this goal encourages self-reproach.

The use of a phrase such as "war on poverty"—calling as it does either for winning or losing—leaves no room for mixed outcomes which inevitably become associated with failure. The poor are still with us. Our programs succeed in reducing their number and their suffering but do not eliminate poverty. And trying just isn't good enough for Americans. Vince Lombardi's view of the importance of winning is deeply rooted in our collective psyche. Social welfare programs born of a reformist spirit and put in place to solve problems will always be susceptible to the charge of failure in a nation as enamored with success as ours. Since we expect our programs to provide permanent solutions, when poverty increases because of poor economic conditions (as during the 1970s and 1980s), we do not consider how much worse the increase in poverty would have been without the programs in place. Instead, we use the data on increased poverty to support accusations that the programs are ineffective—or worse, counterproductive. Conditions are never improving fast enough or at a low enough cost. There will always be new problems that existing programs, in the accepted political vernacular, "totally fail" to address.

Yet, America's reformist temperament is hardly a sufficient explanation for the negative tone of contemporary social welfare debates. It is not as if Americans *never* celebrate success, even partial success. We are not *always* hell-bent on reform. "If it ain't broke, don't fix it" is as much a part of our folk wisdom as "There's always room for improvement." We bestow political rewards on both a John F. Kennedy who tells us that we should try harder and a Ronald Reagan who praises our virtue and accomplishment. The propensity to discuss social welfare policy in relentlessly negative terms must spring from deeper roots.

One source is surely the implicit (sometimes explicit) competition between social welfare programs and one of America's guiding social myths—rugged individualism. Thinking about social welfare policy requires one to focus on dependency, on needs, and on the risks facing members of any society. Such policies achieve, therefore, the usual popularity of messengers with unwelcome news. They remind us constantly that the image of Americans as heroic architects of their own individual fates is something of a fantasy. We cannot quite forgive the social welfare "safety net" for suggesting that we might need it, that we are vulnerable, even mortal.

Yet this explanation also seems insufficient. Our exaltation of rugged individualism coexists with a celebration of family and community solidarity. The barn raising metaphor for good neighborliness still portrays a compelling aspiration. Celebra-

4

tion of private acts of charity is ubiquitous, as are the charitable organizations that channel and publicize efforts to improve the lives of the less fortunate and the life of the community generally. When George Bush spoke of a "kinder, gentler America" and "a thousand points of light," he was elected, not laughed off the ballot. Rugged individualism is not our only defining ideal.

Nevertheless, a focus on the individual and individualism points generally in the right direction. The negative image of American social welfare policy has much to do with our most basic ideas of individual-state relations. Our idea of the good or legitimate state is in conflict with the idea of the state—the *welfare* state—that social welfare programs both create and define. There are several elements in this interpretation.

First, to pursue the welfare of any society is to pursue policies thought to better the lives of individuals. Enhancing individuals' lives is of course a laudable aim, but does it necessarily entail a *state* commitment? Since there are virtually boundless possibilities for increasing individual satisfaction, the activities that might be justified in the name of welfare are similarly limitless. The welfare state accordingly challenges the adequacy, even the legitimacy, of the liberal (or limited) state. In a polity where state is equated with government, and where liberty is equated with limited government, it is easy to regard the welfare state as a threat to liberty.

Second, because government action is commonly viewed as threatening individual liberty, state action to promote *social* welfare can be portrayed as threatening *individual* welfare. A citizen dependent on the state is not free from it, but entangled with it. Moreover, this entanglement has a vastly different social and political significance than being embedded in a family or a community. Although mutually supportive, family and community ties also cultivate individual competence and reinforce individual responsibility. These are dependencies, we are told, that strengthen individual capacities for independence from the state, an independence viewed as crucial to individual welfare. Dependence on the state, in contrast, erodes self-respect and undermines individual capacities.

Finally, by supplementing or supplanting familial and private arrangements for increasing group welfare, social welfare programs challenge these highly valued institutions. To substitute the state for individual, family, community, or other responsible institutions seems to discourage them and to weaken the market and social arrangements for which they are essential. Because American political ideology does not identify the state with society or with nongovernment institutions, the *responsible* state can easily imply *irresponsible* citizens. Accordingly, any generalized commitment to the welfare state appears as a commitment to a self-evidently bad idea—the erosion and eventual destruction of the substate associational arrangements that form the backbone of American society.

Viewed in this way, it is not hard to see why the "welfare state" label, if used at all, is typically pejorative in American political parlance, employed not to describe or explain social welfare arrangements, but to attack their legitimacy. To talk about the welfare state, welfare programs, or even social welfare policy is, from this perspective, to engage a subject that is at least slightly disreputable.

Yet the explanation remains incomplete. Just as our tendency to be hypercritical is balanced by a love of self-celebration, and our individualistic ethos by a celebration of community, so the American public's fear of government is counterbalanced by a strong tradition of looking to government, especially the federal government, as a protector of individual liberty. To be sure, antitrust activities, consumer protection legislation, the setting of minimum labor standards, and the enforcement of antidiscrimination statutes are for some liberty-threatening interventions. But the vast majority of Americans regard government activism of this sort as necessary to protect individual freedom from private abuse. The civil rights movement, we should recall, demanded positive government action in the name of freedom.

Hence, although individual freedom is probably the most cherished of all American values, abusive government is not seen as the only barrier to its enjoyment. When the public feels threatened by private agglomerations of power or by impersonal market forces, it turns to the government for protection. When President Franklin Roosevelt said in his State of the Union message in 1944 that "necessitous men are not free men," he had in mind the American understanding that market forces could coerce just as powerfully as governments could.[7]

The American public's love of freedom need not inevitably translate into distrust of the welfare state. Indeed, despite the negative tone of so much public debate concerning American social welfare policy in the 1970s and 1980s, most of the programs that comprise the American welfare state enjoy strong public support. Such approval would be incomprehensible if most Americans regarded them only as liberty-threatening or otherwise illegitimate.[8] It seems more likely that the public views many welfare state programs as liberty-enhancing, at least when considered in isolation rather than in the context of tirades against big government.

A more compelling account of the negativism of American public discourse about social welfare is needed. Our critical temperament, individualistic self-image, and preference for limited government do help explain our public susceptibility to negative assessment of the welfare state. There are strings in the American heart that critics of the welfare state can pluck. But why have antistate musicians played so fervently since the mid-1970s? And why has the public been so responsive to their efforts? The answers undoubtedly lie in the economy's poor performance and the accompanying sense of national disintegration.

DISAPPOINTED DREAMS

The economic story is easily told. From the end of the Second World War until the early 1970s, the American economy delivered steadily increasing material rewards. Since then, our expectations of continued improvements in living standards have been dealt a series of severe shocks. A quadrupling of oil prices in 1973–74 was followed by the most severe recession since the 1930s. The recovery that followed was soured by spiraling inflation rates. A second oil shock in 1979 prompted an even worse recession. A long recovery began in 1982, but high unemployment and an increasing gap between the wealthiest and the poorer segments of society, accentuated by the growth of highly visible social problems, continue to undermine the public's sense of well-being. Although the 1980s were a generally happier period in the economic and social life of the nation than the 1970s, we remain apprehensive about our future economic performance and particularly about our capacity to deal with the urban decay that both saddens and threatens us.

The sense that things are not going well has not been based on surface impressions alone. From 1947 until 1973 American families enjoyed a long period of steadily rising income. In 1947 median family income (expressed in 1987 dollars) was $15,422. Over the next quarter-century, it increased at an average annual rate of almost 3 percent, standing at $30,820 in 1973. Since then the trend has gone flat, holding roughly steady during the rest of the 1970s, declining in the recession of the early 1980s, and returning to its 1973 level only in 1987, when it stood at $30,853 (see figure 1.1).[9]

It is also worth noting the trend toward greater income inequality since 1973. The poorest 20 percent of the population living in families experienced a 10.8 percent decline in their average real income from 1973 to 1987, with almost all of that decline occurring since 1979. Over the same period, the richest

20 percent of the population living in families experienced a 24.1 percent increase in their average real income. For families with children, the shift toward greater inequality has been even more pronounced.[10]

There have been other, more palpable, signs of economic trouble. Both inflation and unemployment rose to levels well above those of the earlier postwar period. Between 1948 and 1973, the nation's unemployment rate averaged 4.8 percent; since 1973 it has averaged 7.2 percent. The inflation rate averaged 2.7 percent over the earlier period and 6.8 percent since 1973. These two measures of economic dysfunction are often added together to construct a "misery index" indicating the

Figure 1.1 Median Family Income,[a] 1947 to 1987
(1987 dollars, thousands)

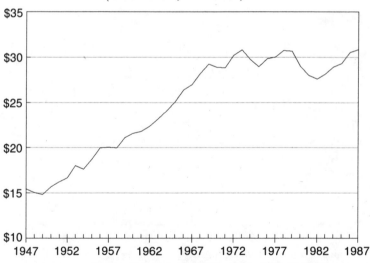

SOURCE: *Current Population Reports*, Series P-60, No. 162.
[a]Includes all households of two or more persons residing together who are related by birth, marriage, or adoption.

combined impact of unemployment and inflation on peoples' lives. Between 1948 and 1973, the so-called misery index averaged 7.5 percent. Since then it has averaged 14 percent (see figure 1.2).

At the same time, the steady progress we had been making in reducing poverty came to an end. Between 1950 and 1973, the proportion of the nation's population living in families with incomes below the poverty line declined by almost two-thirds, from about 30 percent to 11.1 percent. Since then, the poverty rate has edged back up to 13.5 percent (see figure 1.3). For younger, middle-class Americans, the standard dream of owning their own homes became a nightmare of escalating prices and interest rates combined with stagnating earnings. The less

Figure 1.2   Misery Index,[a] 1948 to 1988

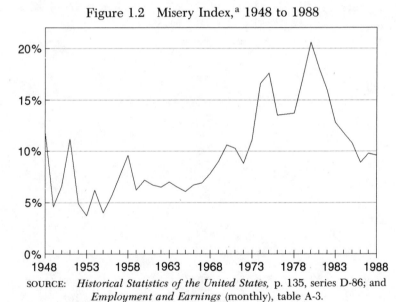

SOURCE: *Historical Statistics of the United States,* p. 135, series D-86; and *Employment and Earnings* (monthly), table A-3.

[a]Annual unemployment rate added to annual rate of inflation of Consumer Price Index

fortunate, during the same period, added a major new category to our lexicon of social ills—homelessness.

Given the economic disappointments experienced by the American public since the early 1970s, it is hardly surprising that charges of failure and crisis in the welfare state have found a ready audience. It is also understandable that large segments of the population would believe those who claim that the welfare state produced the nation's economic problems. All of us know the appeal of the causal fallacy, *post hoc, ergo propter hoc.* The period preceding the onset of stagflation in the American economy was presented as a liberal heyday in which generous

Figure 1.3   Official Poverty Rate, 1948 to 1987

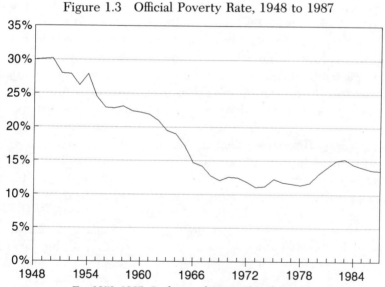

SOURCE: For 1959–1987, *Background Material and Data on Programs within the Jurisdiction of the Committee on Ways and Means,* Committee Print, 1989, p. 944, table 2. For 1948–1958, data extrapolated from *Economic Report of the President* (January 1969), p. 154, chart 10.

11

social policies ran rampant. The Johnson administration advertised its commitment to a war on poverty, and a bevy of new programs was indeed inaugurated. Social welfare expenditures did rise dramatically, though not because of the war on poverty.

A survey of newspaper articles on the Great Society covering the period 1968 to 1988 reveals an evolving pattern of commentary. During the first phase, from roughly 1969 to 1975, complaints tended to focus on administrative difficulties and fiscal concerns. The fiscal attacks continued into the second phase (roughly 1974 to 1979) but were joined by the growing sentiment that Great Society programs had caused the economic difficulties of the mid-1970s and that dismantling them was serving the antipoverty cause. From 1980 until about 1984, the causative link between the Great Society programs and the problems they were meant to correct became even more direct. The message of conservative critics like George Gilder was repeatedly echoed by President Reagan in his first term, and finally by Charles Murray in *Losing Ground.*[11]

It was easy to blame the expansion in the welfare state for the stagflation that followed, easier still to view the war on poverty and the programmatic embodiments of the Great Society as failures and our expanded welfare state as teetering on collapse. We shall see that each of these claims is false, but it is not surprising that those skeptical about America's social welfare programs disproportionately shaped—in tone and in substance—the nation's perception of its social problems and the capacity of American government to ameliorate them. The time was ripe for an attack on the welfare state based on that portion of national political ideology that emphasized individual, family, voluntary associations, and market as bulwarks against government profligacy and the erosion of freedom.

A CHORUS OF CRITICS

Conservative critics of the welfare state were quick to take advantage of the American public's unease. They worked over-time to convince Americans that social welfare spending was at the root of the country's economic and social problems, but little of what they said was really new. Indeed, critics of the New Deal had made the same arguments in the 1930s. Federal social welfare programs threaten the economy's long-term health by withdrawing productive resources from the private sector through taxation and borrowing. Economic prosperity, the only genuine means of overcoming poverty, is deferred as we apply well-meaning but counterproductive nostrums to the nation's social problems. By burdening our children with debt and transfer obligations, we rob them of a future and make it all the more difficult for them to correct our mistakes. These wrong-headed policies guarantee that worsening crises are in-evitable in our economic future. When they come, our children will not even be able to enjoy the seemingly beneficial effects of the social programs we have set in place; they will no longer be able to afford them. In the meantime, the lot of the poor will grow worse as the welfare state saps them of initiative and self-respect. Their only real hope of escaping poverty, a willing-ness to work hard in their own interest, is being sold for a mess of federal pottage. And worse, we all stand to lose our freedom as, piece by piece, we turn over responsibility for our individual and collective fate to the bureaucrats of big government. It was all said in the 1930s, but in the early 1970s the old arguments were heard again, advanced this time with greater analytical sophistication and renewed zeal.

Ironically, the plausibility of the conservative broadside against the welfare state was enhanced in the 1970s and 1980s by earlier criticism from the left wing of American politics. In the late 1960s and early 1970s, the voice of the American Left was transmitted to the public through the actions of a variety of anti-Establishment protest movements and organizations. The views expressed about the welfare state were generally condemnatory. For example, in their widely read 1971 book, *Regulating the Poor,* Frances Fox Piven and Richard Cloward attacked the moral integrity of public assistance programs. Denying that humanitarian motives or a genuine desire to end poverty had ever played a determinative role in public assistance, Piven and Cloward argued that welfare programs instead functioned as instruments of social control, providing only enough assistance to calm popular unrest among the poor while using work requirements to impose the discipline of the labor-market on them.[12] Note that this argument directly contradicted the conservative portrayal of public assistance; nonetheless arguments on the Left that encouraged a cynical view of antipoverty programs made it easier for conservatives to press their own attacks.

Other left-wing criticism of the welfare state supported conservative positions in more direct ways. In his influential book, *The Fiscal Crisis of the State,* James O'Connor argued that the United States had developed a "warfare/welfare state."[13] According to O'Connor, America's prosperity depended on the imperial power, fiscal stimulus, and social control provided by the combination of its military and social welfare spending. But by the 1970s, American government was losing its capacity to finance the economy's evergrowing needs for both fiscal stimulus and social pacification. Although O'Connor's argument conflicted with key elements of the conservative critique of the welfare state, it supported the conservative view that capitalism cannot afford the welfare state over the long run.

As the protest politics of the 1960s died down in the 1970s, the Left lost its visibility, and left-wing views of the welfare state lost their salience in American public debate. The field of battle was occupied more prominently by conservative jousters, but the legacy of the Left's criticism remained. Liberal defenders of American social welfare policy had been bloodied by their earlier encounter with the Left. Their ideological defenses had been weakened, and they now had to contend with a far stronger challenge from the Right. Liberalism was whipsawed.

The conservative campaign against the American welfare state unfolded on several levels. Academic experts provided scholarly analyses of many social welfare programs and helped formulate the general conservative critique of their aims and performance. A vigorous group of conservative commentators and editors made sure that popularized versions of this scholarship reached decision makers and ultimately the public.

The course of Martin Feldstein's work illustrates this process. President of the National Bureau of Economic Research from 1977 to 1982, and then chairman of President Reagan's Council of Economic Advisors, Feldstein produced an impressive body of esoteric research arguing that the Social Security financing system has a substantial, negative effect on the economy's savings rate.[14] Originally published in journals read only by scholars, his conclusions were widely disseminated in the daily press and in magazines oriented to public issues. Eventually his contentions filtered through to the general public in the form of generalized charges that Social Security was strangling the economy. More recent research has largely discredited Feldstein's argument, as we shall see in chapter 5's discussion of Social Security. The effect of Feldstein's writing on public perceptions of Social Security has nevertheless been substantial. Scholarly criticism of the conservative attack on the welfare state was extensive, but, as usual, the scholarly review never caught up with the dissemination in the media of the original attacks.

In similar fashion, the work of a growing fraternity of conservative writers reached a public distraught over the state of the economy. Financial support for both conservative scholarship and the dissemination of conservative policy analysis burgeoned in the 1970s. At the beginning of the decade, the American Enterprise Institute was a small think tank with a staff of 19 and a budget of less than $900,000. By 1980 it had a staff of 135 and a budget of $10.4 million. The Heritage Foundation, established in 1973, grew at an annual rate of 40 percent a year for the next decade. Its budget was $7.1 million in the 1981–82 fiscal year.[15] A host of less well-known conservative research institutes and foundations were also established, and funding for older conservative think tanks like the Hoover Institution increased substantially.

Those who financed this growth were clear about their aims. They sought to increase the flow of conservative scholarship directly into American intellectual life and political debate. The strategy appears to have been effective. Scholars like Milton Friedman became minor media celebrities, gurus of a self-confident and seemingly authoritative conservatism. American social welfare policy became regularly a topic of castigation and condescending scorn. Liberal defenders of the welfare state seemed tired, overwhelmed by American conservatism's newly amplified voice.[16]

And so, from at least the mid-1970s, the dialogue on social welfare policy has run primarily to handwringing and teeth gnashing. Moreover, the conclusions of many of the most visible attempts to evaluate American social welfare policy seem to coalesce: American social welfare policies and programs are economically, socially, or morally bankrupt. In the press, the major opinion and newsmagazines, and the most widely discussed books on the subject, American social welfare provision has been most often characterized as ungovernable, unaffordable, or undesirable—sometimes all three at once.

If these claims were correct, we would have to agree that the American welfare state is a disaster, that our current collection of programs had better be dismantled, and the sooner the better. Moreover, if the ungovernability charge is to be believed, we are helpless. The broad public support for the largest social

16

welfare programs is dismaying evidence of the well-entrenched interests created by the welfare state that now surround it and make major social policy reform virtually impossible. In this view, the seemingly cheerful news from the opinion polls that Americans overwhelmingly approve of our major social welfare programs at best tells us that we are going to hell in a handbasket we like. The pleasures of this journey are unlikely to console us, however, once we reach the destination.

IDEOLOGY FROM THE GROUND UP

It should be apparent by now that the American welfare state is laboring under severe political disadvantages. First, it is subject to ideological misgivings of a distinctively American type. Second, its growth has become identified, since the 1973–74 oil crisis, with a period of relative economic stagnation. Finally, it has been the target of a well-organized and exceedingly articulate campaign of conservative criticism.

Yet, having recognized all this, we are not prepared to accept the presumption that the American welfare state is ungovernable, unaffordable, or undesirable. Surely it is possible to admit that social welfare programs in the United States bear special burdens of justification without simultaneously conceding that such programs must inevitably be viewed as problems, failures, or embarrassments. After all, a part of America's ideological heritage is that "ideology," as such, should not get in the way of problem solving. We have in fact built up a complex of social programs that elsewhere would, without pejorative inflection, be called a welfare state. Having done that, there must be some way that we can learn to talk about what we have wrought without undue and reflexive handwringing.

One way to move toward rhetorical neutrality is to be specific, to talk about concrete problems in particular programs, ignoring, as much as possible, the symbolic significance of what

17

is happening. In this way, we focus on old-age pensions, medical care, child poverty, or the problems of the disabled, to take but a few examples. This is, indeed, the pattern of most social welfare talk in the United States, and it will be the pattern of much of ours in this volume. The values of this approach as an operational strategy are both immense and obvious.

But there are disadvantages as well to this kind of discussion. The social policy dialogue fragments into technical subspecialties. In that process the overarching connections among programs are lost and the general public, even the attentive observer of government policy, is left baffled about what is really going on. The fragmentation of issues encourages the ubiquitous complaint that our social welfare efforts are a "crazy quilt" of overlapping and conflicting programs that both waste resources and leave large gaps in coverage. In addition, program-by-program analyses, because they inevitably become highly technical, promote a sense of disenfranchisement, the feeling that social welfare policy is the province of specialists who may not care much about the public's real political desires.

Moreover, the failure to talk about overall social welfare policy creates or exacerbates other misunderstandings. For example, continuous political concern about morally controversial programs such as Aid to Families with Dependent Children (AFDC) is not tempered by an appreciation of the very special, and fiscally very limited, place such programs occupy in the American welfare state. The result is a general sense of malaise that attaches to a broad range of programs having quite different purposes, structures, and effects. Similarly, talk about huge levels of social welfare spending in general is confused with much smaller levels of expenditure for "welfare" or "poverty" programs. Huge outlays then seem, somehow, not to be solving a relatively smaller "poverty" problem. The impression given is again one of massive waste or mismanagement—an impression that can be countered only by a more general understanding of how our social welfare expenditures are, in fact, struc-

tured and why that structure is congruent with political purposes that are widely shared among nearly every group in the
American polity.

THE PLAN OF THIS BOOK

Our first task, then, in confronting the massive misunderstanding and the relentlessly negative coloration of American social
policy discourse, is to come to terms with our ideological heritage. We need to understand what we have done, but more
important, we need to understand our acts in appropriate symbolic terms. In chapter 2 we see how the United States can have
almost all the programmatic features of a mature welfare state
while regarding "welfare statism" with suspicion. To see this it
is necessary to understand the general features of peculiarly
American political commitments. It is also necessary to understand something of our history and something about our possible futures. Our ideology is embedded at least as deeply in what
we do as in what we say. And when looking at what we do, a
striking and coherent philosophy of our social welfare provision
emerges.

Chapter 3 provides a more detailed description of American
social welfare programs and a more policy-analytic explanation
of why the American welfare state has been so widely regarded
as critically troubled. The basic story is quite straightforward.
This is not the 1950s or the 1960s; economic realities, demographic characteristics, and political perceptions have shifted.
The questions of concern are equally straightforward. Has the
welfare state kept pace with these developments? In what
ways? If not, or to the extent it has not, what does that portend
for the future? Can we afford to continue our prior commitments? Can we change, even if we want to?

We then take a more disaggregated look at three of the
American welfare state's major program areas: welfare, Social

Security pensions, and medical care. We have chosen this programmatic focus for chapters 4 through 6 for several reasons. First, some specificity is necessary if we are to understand concretely the strengths and weaknesses of our current complex of programs. Second, except for general public education, these three domains account for the bulk of welfare state expenditures. Finally, welfare, pensions, and medical care illustrate, respectively, the three main categories of charges against the current configuration of the American welfare state—undesirability, ungovernability, and unaffordability.

We have indicated already our belief that these charges are unfounded. Indeed, we will argue that, in the one domain where they most apply, medical care, the criticisms are appropriate only because of a major *gap* in welfare state provision, not because of the "bankruptcy" of our social welfare programs. The discussion of medical care thus presents a necessary elaboration of chapter 2's restricted claim about the coherence of America's welfare state. We do not argue that America has in place *all* the social welfare programs that would be compatible with the nation's constant commitments, only that the major features of our most substantial programs are *compatible* with our relatively stable post–New Deal political ideology.

Beyond setting the record straight, we also want to call attention to a common set of fallacies that underlie many contemporary stories of social welfare gloom and doom. These fallacies make most of the critical stories both simple and attractive and their rebuttal both complex and painful. Our hope is that, by illustration and analysis of common analytic failures, we can induce our readers to adopt a reflexive skepticism when confronted with certain varieties of unhelpful social welfare policy talk. We fear that only by developing the ability to spot the likely policy-analytic blunder *before* having the evidence with which to refute it can concerned citizens protect themselves in a policy dialogue that too often features nonsense in place of sense. Chapter 7 focuses on these patterns of analytic failure and their antidotes.

The chapter's title—"How Not to Think about the American Welfare State"—bluntly illustrates our concern with misunderstandings about American social welfare policy. But concentrating on what is *not* wrong with American social policy is an incomplete agenda. We must be able to see both what is right and what is wrong, what the welfare state actually has done and what it can do, and what its real purposes and effects have been. To do so means appreciating the importance of ideology in shaping American social policy. That in turn requires thinking about social programs and their reform from the standpoint of the ideology the programs really express and the limits on reform that our ideological history imposes.

2

::

The American Opportunity-Insurance State

Perhaps no critique of social welfare program performance is more ubiquitous than that which imagines programs to have single purposes that have somehow been lost in their implementation. A common example of this critical myopia is the assumption that reducing poverty is the central aim of American social welfare policy. The usual form of this argument begins by assuming that any program under discussion—Social Security, AFDC, Food Stamps, Unemployment Insurance (UI)—is (or should be) directed toward the alleviation of poverty. All fail to do so, or fail to do so completely, or also support the non-poor. Why? Because they serve other, non-poverty purposes as well. Now here is the crucial juncture in the argument. The critic then concludes that reform is required to make the program structure fit the antipoverty objective. Depending on the critic's political proclivity and the particular program under discussion, the policy favored can be stricter means testing, increased benefits, "cashing out" in-kind supplements, and so on.

But this is to go much too far, much too fast. Even more, it is wrong-headed or, sometimes, simply wrong. The appropriate response to the initial criticism is to ask, "So what?" Does the critic think society's *only* purpose is to eliminate poverty? If not, should social welfare programs be structured as if that were our only goal? If not, what is wrong with the other goals served by the program now under discussion? And so on. Only after the third question is reached can useful policy analysis proceed.

CONCEPTIONS OF PURPOSE

There are, indeed, at least four fundamental conceptions of purpose that coexist, often uneasily, in the design of American social welfare programs. Each embodies a distinct ideological vision of the welfare state and tends to be preferred by certain political actors and interest groups. We term the four visions "behaviorist," "residualist," "social insurance," and "populist." In designing new programs or in revising old ones, these visions compete with one another. Compromise results. Call it contradiction if you wish. One purpose may dominate the others in a particular program, or it may be eclipsed entirely, but ambiguity is far more common than clarity. Conflict between purposes is unavoidable. To aspire to a welfare state that is free of such inconsistencies is to reject political and social complexity.

Behaviorist. The behaviorist vision of social welfare policy has deep historical roots in the English poor law system that preceded the modern welfare state. According to this view, social welfare policy is mainly concerned with the task of inducing the poor to behave in a more socially acceptable manner. The able-bodied should work at whatever jobs are available. Families should assume responsibility for the care of the young, the old, and the disabled. Everyone should look to their own future, providing for both expected and unexpected reductions in earning power. If the poor conformed their behavior to this ideal, social welfare programs could limit their activities to charitable relief for victims of truly exceptional circumstance. Indeed, private charity might reasonably be expected to perform this task without the assistance of the state. The poor are poor—and suffer from a lack of medical care, food, housing, and security—because they do not live as they should. The most basic sense of humaneness requires that such suffering be partially relieved. But generous assistance would reinforce the very behavior patterns that cause the suffering in the first place.

In particular, public assistance should generally be denied when the behavior at issue is immediately correctable, as with the able-bodied poor who need only submit themselves to the discipline of the labor market. Long-term assistance may be necessary when the behavior at issue has moved past correction, as with elderly paupers lacking both family and savings. The assistance provided in any case should be marginal, even punitive, in order to discourage fraudulent appeals for help and to deliver a message to the nonelderly about the importance of conforming.

One of the most vivid illustrations of the behaviorist attitude can be found in the writings of the pessimistic demographer and economist Thomas Malthus. He argued that poverty is the predictable result of individual decisions to marry and have children when wage levels are insufficient to support a family.

When the wages of labour are hardly sufficient to maintain two children, a man marries and has five or six; he of course finds himself miserably distressed. He accuses the insufficiency of the price of labour to maintain a family. He accuses his parish for their tardy and sparing fulfillment of their obligation to assist him. He accuses the avarice of the rich, who suffer him to want what they can so well spare. He accuses the partial and unjust institutions of society, which have awarded him an inadequate share of the produce of the earth. He accuses perhaps the dispensations of providence, which have assigned to him a place in society so beset with unavoidable distress and dependence. In searching for objects of accusation, he never adverts to the quarter from which his misfortunes originate. The last person that he would think of accusing is himself, on whom in fact the principal blame lies, except so far as he has been deceived by the higher classes of society.[1]

Malthus condemned the poor laws, and even private charity, for "removing from each individual that heavy responsibility, which he would incur by the laws of nature, for bringing beings into the world which he could not support."[2]

This point of view has considerable contemporary expression. Modern behaviorists like Charles Murray concern themselves with a broader range of suspect behaviors, but they share with Malthus the generalized suspicion that by supporting the poor and therefore encouraging dependency, the welfare state does more harm than good. Behaviorists are among the welfare state's most ardent and uncompromising critics; they also concern themselves with the design of specific social welfare programs. Their point of view is reflected, for instance, in the almost complete exclusion from the American welfare state of programs providing cash assistance to persons considered employable and in the consuming concern for work incentives apparent in the structure of most means-tested antipoverty programs.

Residualist. The view of the welfare state that we term residualist trades on the metaphor of the "safety net." The net of social welfare programs in this view is intended to rescue the victims of capitalism and to give subsistence level relief to those unable to provide for their own needs. This view of purpose also grew out of the English poor law tradition, but it more nearly reflects the legacy of philanthropic humanitarianism in that tradition than the influence of the workhouse disciplinarian. It is found virtually everywhere among capitalist nations, though its popularity varies enormously. In the United States, and in Australia and Canada as well, this residualist conception is the staple not only of business and financial elites, but of large numbers of middle- and lower-income people as well.

Most of those who think of the welfare state as "residual" believe that its aim should be temporary assistance and its administration highly decentralized. They aspire to a system in

which the distribution of "relief" is closely supervised by offi-
cials who are thoroughly familiar with the circumstances of
their clients' lives, thereby ensuring that only the "deserving"
poor receive assistance. In federal regimes the diffusion of authority for social programs to states and provinces has been a
rallying cry of residualists. In the United States, public assistance programs such as the federal-state Aid to Dependent
Children (now Aid to Families with Dependent Children,
AFDC), which was part of the original Social Security Act of
1935, exemplify this ideal. In Canada similar developments
took place, reinforced with constitutional requirements that
the provinces be responsible for social programs except as provided by constitutional amendment.[3] Advocacy of decentraliza-
tion presumes that individual families will typically assure the
welfare of their members. When that fails, institutions close to
those families—charitable groups, then local and provincial or
state programs—constitute the safety net protecting against
destitution.

The metaphor of the safety net suggests the key features of
appropriate welfare policy. The net is close to the ground and
the benefits are accordingly modest—a subsistence that might
well vary widely in connection with community standards of
adequacy. The clientele are the down and out; the eligibility
criteria are designed to sort out the truly needy from the rest.
There is here an implicit notion of potential waste that it is
important to avoid: aid to those who do not need it. Minimal
adequacy, selectivity, localism, and tests of need—these constitute the residualist's standard bases for evaluating the welfare
state.

Social Insurance. Residualism of this type sharply differs
from what we term the social insurance model of the welfare
state. The basic purpose of the welfare state, according to this
view, is to provide economic security, to prevent people from
falling into destitution rather than rescuing them after they

have already fallen. The aim is something like the universaliza-
tion of the financial security presumed in the fringe benefits of
higher civil servants and economic elites. The threats to economic security include some obvious ones—involuntary unemployment, widowhood, sickness, injury, or retirement—as well
as some less obvious ones such as a large family. Welfare states
have provided for these eventualities at different times, in different sequences, and with considerable variation in generosity
and terms of administration.[4] Yet, irrespective of the form and
level of payment, social insurance programs have rejected as
inferior the selective machinery of means-tested programs: The
more universal are both contributions and benefits, the closer
the program is to the social insurance model.

The central image of social insurance is the earned entitlement, publicly administered benefits for which all similarly situ-
ated persons are eligible by virtue of their financial contributions to the system or the taxes they pay. Sometimes the
contributions are made in the form of general tax payments, as
is partly the case in Canada. Or contributions may take the form
of flat payments for social insurance, as was the case in Britain
until the 1970s. Or special proportional taxes may be designated for the system's support, as with the familiar FICA (Federal Insurance Contributions Act) payroll tax in the United
States. Whatever the arrangement, the idea is to contribute
while working to protection when out of work. Equitable treatment, not the equalizing of incomes, is the controlling standard.

The redistribution of income is clearly one consequence of
such programs, but it is not their primary aim. And the model
of redistribution is not so much intended to be between
socioeconomic classes as over the life cycle of individuals and
their families. The relevant question for the proponents of social insurance involves the adequacy of the citizenry's preparation for the predictable risks of modern industrial society.
Looked at this way, *social* insurance simply extends the security
aims of private insurance to circumstances where either the

risks are uninsurable privately or the purchase of adequate levels of commercial insurance is unlikely.

Such a broad characterization is bound to miss the details of one or another nation's mix of programs. No nation has only social insurance programs; everywhere behaviorist, residualist, and social insurance strategies are mixed in the actual range of programs. But variation and mixture do not preclude recognition of the evaluative differences in the perspectives. In the answers to questions about who gets what, when, and where, it makes considerable difference whether the standard is the appropriate inducement to elicit desirable modifications in behavior, appropriate levels of assistance for the destitute, or adequate compensation for losses of earning power.[5]

Egalitarian Populist. So far we have not mentioned the redistribution of wealth and power in our discussion of welfare states. In the behaviorist model, the powerful correct the faults of the weak. In the residualist model, the powerful take care of the weak. Social insurance provides a measure of economic security to the entire population but does not attempt directly to transform power relations in society. From a more egalitarian perspective, the goals of behavior modification, charity, and insurance compensation are viewed as either repressive or inadequate. They constitute adjustments to the harsh realities of industrial society, rather than means for transforming it.

The aim of the egalitarian populist theorist is social change, not guaranteeing insurance payments or providing a safety net for the poor, and certainly not correcting the alleged misbehavior of the poor. The approved means are not ameliorative social programs, but the redistribution of income and power to the less privileged. What social insurance advocates count as generous provision is, for the most critical egalitarian populist, illusory, a way to gloss over the contradictions of modern capitalism.

Theorists of this persuasion have not produced a metaphor

that competes with the disciplinary poorhouse, the safety net, or the earned entitlement. But the images of participatory democracy or the egalitarian collective suggest the aspirational difference. The aim of programs by the people, not for the people, expresses the compelling notion. And that means a rejection of the charitable societies as well as the harsh administrators of the dole, of the Social Security office as well as of the "helping" professions. Bureaucratic professionalism and paternalism alike evoke the wrath of the egalitarian populist, as well as some social democratic reformers who have grown weary of the routines and restraints of mature welfare states.

The egalitarian populist vision of social transformation has been much less influential in the design of the major transfer programs of the American welfare state than the other three perspectives we have identified. But it has not been totally absent. Part of the antipoverty strategy of the 1960s involved efforts to organize the poor to shape the economic and social development of their own communities. There are community development corporations that still aspire to this goal. The financing of legal services for the poor can also be understood as a populist effort to give a measure of "power to the people." Moreover, if we had defined the welfare state more broadly, including, for example, labor relations policy, public education, and progressive taxation, then the influence of egalitarian populist thought would be more evident. In public education particularly, the United States was a leader rather than a laggard in introducing strongly egalitarian principles.

The United States does not have a welfare state that can be characterized consistently in terms of any of the four relatively coherent welfare state ideologies we have identified. Nor in fact does any other nation, although a number come closer to the social insurance model than does the United States. To the extent that commentators on social welfare policy subscribe to one or another of these ideologies, they will find the American welfare state inadequate. Our welfare state goes considerably beyond what behaviorists and residualists think appropriate for state provision. Yet, it has failed to develop programs that carry out the complete logic of social insurance, and it shows very little inclination to move toward some more thoroughly egalitarian vision of the distribution of wealth and power. From each well-established ideological tradition, therefore, the American welfare state seems open to criticism.

Moreover, because social welfare discussion—indeed all political discussion—in the United States tends to avoid ideological elaboration, most of the criticism centers superficially on the means for implementing apparently agreed-on goals. The American welfare state is said to have failed us by not wiping out the scourge of poverty, by not protecting all citizens against cataclysmic medical expense, and by not eliminating the bureaucratic barriers to full participation by needy populations. It is also said to be wasteful, "contradictory," and oppressive. Indeed, as we shall see, the American welfare state is said to have failed us in many other respects as well, ways that this book characterizes as "unaffordable," "undesirable," and "ungovernable."

What is not generally noticed, however, is that these criticisms often proceed from assumptions about purpose that make sense within one ideological framework but not others. Hence, it is not just that the American welfare state has failed to fulfill any particular ideological preference. Rather, the discussions of the American welfare state that are divorced from specification of the ideological perspective of the discussants tend to conflate criticisms of purpose with criticisms of practices or effects. All the commentators can be seen to be unhappy. What is more difficult to see is that they typically confuse the pursuit of an alternative purpose with a failure to achieve their own favorite welfare state goals.

This situation is perhaps not critical in a polity in which government actors are continuously about the business of explaining and justifying programmatic activity in terms of national goals. But, since the administration of Lyndon Johnson, there have been few champions of any particular vision of American social welfare policy who have taken it on themselves to explain how that vision is and is not being realized by the current complex of social welfare programs. From the partial retreat from state activism of the Nixon, Ford, and Carter administrations, to the almost complete abandonment of the idea of the state as a solution to social problems during the Reagan years to George Bush's "thousand points of light," we have been treated to a political dialogue with an essential ingredient missing. We have programs, but we seem not to have any principles. And, in the absence of continuous attempts to articulate policy in terms of principle, public understanding is almost certain to be lost.

CORE COMMITMENTS

In the jumble of seemingly contradictory goals that have shaped the design of the American welfare state, we believe a more or less coherent set of enduring commitments can be discerned. The income transfer programs we actually have created tend to fall into one of two categories. They either insure broad strata of the nation's population against impoverishment from the loss of a breadwinner's income, or they assist those whom opportunity has passed by. In other words, what has emerged from our ongoing squabbles over the proper goals of social welfare policy is a set of programs that can be described with a fair degree of accuracy as constituting not so much a welfare state as an "insurance/opportunity state."

Social Insurance. Social welfare expenditures in the United States consist overwhelmingly of social insurance payments. The total amount spent by all levels of government for social insurance benefits is illustrated, using data for 1986, in table 2.1.

Table 2.1   Social Insurance Expenditures, 1986

	Beneficiaries (thousands)	Benefits (Millions of Dollars)
TOTAL	(NA)	$360,073
Federal[a]	(NA)	307,361
State[a]	(NA)	52,712
Social Security Benefits	37,703	269,724
Retirement	26,541	140,418
Disability	3,995	19,524
Survivors	7,166	33,785
Medicare	31,750[b]	75,997
Public Employee Retirement[c]	7,098	37,431
Railroad Retirement[d]	960	6,418
Unemployment Insurance[e]	2,415[f]	18,678
Workers' Compensation	(NA)	24,382
Other Programs[g]	(NA)	3,440

SOURCE: *Statistical Abstract of the United States* (1989), tables 566, 571, 579, 594.

[a] Estimate

[b] Enrolled

[c] Estimated Social Security equivalent payments for retirement, disability, and survivors benefits.

[d] Includes old age, survivors, and disability benefits.

[e] Includes compensation for federal employees and ex-servicemen, trade adjustment and cash training allowance, railroad unemployment insurance, and payments under extended, emergency, disaster, and special unemployment insurance programs.

[f] Includes only regular state unemployment insurance, ex-servicemen program, and railroad unemployment insurance beneficiaries.

[g] Includes Black Lung Benefit Program and state temporary disability benefits payable in CA, NJ, NY, RI, and PR.

The picture does not change much from year to year. The principal beneficiaries of our social insurance programs are the elderly. Social Security old-age pensions alone account for about 39 percent of all social insurance payments, and Medicare benefits for predominantly the same population account for another 21 percent. Old-age pensions for government and rail-road workers account for almost 10 percent more of the total.[6] And the great bulk of the $360.1 billion in benefits (about 85 percent) was provided by the federal government, mostly in the form of Social Security payments.

The basic outline of America's social insurance programs was developed in 1935 in a remarkable document: *The Report of the Committee on Economic Security.*[7] The committee, consisting of four cabinet secretaries and the director of the New Deal's public relief effort, was appointed by President Franklin Roosevelt to propose to him programs that would provide "some safeguard against misfortunes which cannot be wholly eliminated in this man-made world of ours."[8] In 1935 the insecurity created by those misfortunes was all too apparent.

The committee quickly concluded two things. "The one almost all-embracing measure of security" was, in the committee's mind, "an assured income."[9] But assurance of income divorced from productivity was emphatically not the idea behind the committee's proposals. Instead, the central conception was to ensure that every employable person would have the opportunity to be self-supporting—through public employment if the private sector failed to provide enough jobs—while developing transfer programs that would deal with the hazards that made the continuous receipt of income through productive work problematic for many, if not most, Americans during some stage of their life. Those hazards included illness, disability, old age, or the loss of the support of a father or husband. And, as the Depression had made graphic for tens of millions, even those in their most productive years and unimpaired by illness or disability might be thrown out of work by the impersonal forces of the market.

Although the Report of the Committee on Economic Security was notable for its programmatic initiatives, it was much more important for its political and philosophical underpinnings. The committee concentrated relentlessly on economic opportunity as the primary basis for individual support. The report emphasized public stimulation of job creation and public employment as the preferred means of delivering public assistance to the long-term unemployed (unemployment insurance cash payments were proposed then, and remain now, available for quite short periods of time). It also insisted on a tight link between work and social insurance benefits. Eligibility, whether for unemployment insurance, survivor's benefits, or an old-age pension, depended on prior contributions through taxes on wages. Taxes on productive work both financed the social insurance programs and entitled participants to their protection.

American social insurance is, by virtue of its taxation and benefit schedules, mildly redistributive across groups of workers. But it is not, nor was it ever intended to be, income equalizing in its effects or targeted specifically on the poor. There is no means test for the receipt of payments, and both taxes and benefits are related to, although not directly proportional to, a recipient's prior wages. Social insurance is designed to help families maintain the security they have achieved through productive work.

The committee's proposals for immediate action in this area were limited. The opposition of powerful groups such as the American Medical Association and the insurance industry made the passage of health insurance and disability insurance highly problematic. The committee, therefore, proposed only a program of old-age and survivors' insurance along with a program of unemployment compensation for immediate enactment. Indeed, disability insurance was not added until the mid-1950s; medical insurance did not appear as a national program until 1965, and then only for the aged. American social insurance was conceived whole but implemented incrementally. In terms of its original conception, it is even yet not complete.

The committee's extension of the universalistic principles of social insurance to employment policy was more immediately responsive to the crisis of the Great Depression. To be sure, the committee's proposal that the federal government provide "employment assurance" to the nation's labor force was only partially implemented with the establishment of public employment programs like the Works Progress Administration (WPA) and the advent of Keynesian demand stimulation efforts. Nevertheless, in terms of total spending, this is where the New Deal welfare state placed its greatest emphasis. Between 1933 and 1940, more public money was spent creating jobs for the unemployed in public employment programs than on all other forms of public assistance and social insurance combined. These employment programs were phased out during the Second World War, and they have never been reintroduced on a large scale. Thus, despite its contemporary emphasis on job creation, the New Deal's lasting contribution to the American welfare state was the introduction of large-scale cash transfer programs organized according to social insurance principles.

Means-Tested Programs. The second major component of the American welfare state consists of programs that deliver mainly in-kind assistance to persons who qualify for it on the basis of need. Table 2.2 shows the total amount spent by all levels of government on these programs in 1986.

Several characteristics of these programs are worth noting. First, a comparison of tables 2.1 and 2.2 shows that means-tested aid represents a much smaller part of American social welfare commitments than does social insurance. We spend almost two and a half times as much on social insurance. At the federal level, the disparity is even greater. The federal government spends almost three dollars on social insurance for every dollar spent providing means-tested aid.

Second, relatively little means-tested assistance is provided in the form of cash. In 1986, for instance, cash aid accounted for only 28 percent of all means-tested benefits. Moreover, the amount of cash assistance provided through the two programs that most Americans equate with "welfare," Aid to Families

Table 2.2 Means-Tested Programs, 1986

	Average Monthly Recipients (thousands)	Federal Expenditures ($Millions)	State & Local Expenditures ($Millions)	Total Expenditures ($Millions)
Total	(NA)	108,269	40,436	148,705
Medical				
Benefits	(NA)	29,771	23,226	52,997
Medicaid[a]	22,518	24,767	19,675	44,442
Needy Veterans	361	3,183[b]	—	3,183
General Assistance	(NA)	—	3,259[b]	3,259[b]
Other Medical Care	(NA)	1,821	292	2,113
Cash Aid	(NA)	26,887	14,065	40,952
AFDC[a,c]	10,995	9,536	8,221	17,757
SSI[a,d]	4,450	10,515	2,515	12,823
Pensions for Needy Veterans	1,397[b]	3,874	—	3,874
General Assistance	1,334[b]	—	2,636[b]	2,636[b]
EITC[e]	19,197[b]	2,084	—	2,084
Other Cash Aid	(NA)	1,085	1,080	20,226
Food Benefits				
Food Stamps[a]	20,900	12,529	912	13,441
School Lunch Program	11,600	2,948	—	2,948
WIC[f]	3,312	1,581	—	1,581
Other Food Aid	(NA)	2,088	168	2,256

Table 2.2 (Continued)

	Average Monthly Recipients (thousands)	Federal Expenditures ($Millions)	State & Local Expenditures ($Millions)	Total Expenditures ($Millions)
Housing Benefits	(NA)	13,245	—	13,245
Section 8 Assistance	2,143[g]	7,430	—	7,430
Low Rent Public Housing	1,380[g]	2,882	—	2,882
Other Housing Benefits	(NA)	2,933	—	2,933
Education Aid	(NA)	10,101	488	10,589
Pell Grants	2,881	3,862	—	3,862
Guaranteed Student Loans	3,242	3,288	—	3,288
Head Start	448	1,013	253	1,266
Other Education Assistance	(NA)	1,938	235	2,173
Jobs and Training	(NA)	3,626	73	3,699
Social Services	(NA)	3,390	1,454[b]	4,844[b]
Energy Assistance[a]	(NA)	2,103	50	2,153

SOURCE: U.S. Library of Congress, Congressional Research Service, *Cash and Non-Cash Benefits for Persons with Limited Income: Eligibility Rules, Recipient and Expenditure Data,* FY 1986–88 (24 Oct. 1989), pp. 209–23.

[a] Includes administrative expenses.
[b] Estimated
[c] Aid to Families with Dependent Children
[d] Supplemental Security Income
[e] Earned Income Tax Credit
[f] Special supplemental food program for women, infants, and children.
[g] Units eligible for payment

with Dependent Children and General Assistance, accounted for only half of this total, or 14 percent of all means-tested aid. Instead of cash assistance, most of the help provided to low-income persons in the United States consists of medical care, subsidies for food and housing expenditures, and college tuition assistance. In-kind assistance in these areas accounted for two-thirds of all means-tested aid in 1986. Medical care expenditures alone were responsible for over a third of all means-tested aid provided that year.

Third, state and local governments play a much more important role in the provision of means-tested aid than they do in the provision of social insurance benefits. In 1986, state and local governments accounted for only 15 percent of all social insurance expenditures, and they played a similarly modest role in administering the programs that delivered this aid. The contribution of state and local governments to the financing of means-tested benefits was, in relative terms, almost twice as great, accounting for 27 percent of total expenditures; but they also bore primary responsibility for administering the programs that delivered most of the federal aid as well.

These means-tested programs are often visualized as a residual safety net protecting Americans against complete destitution. However, if ensuring a minimally adequate income for all were the primary focus of American social welfare policy outside the domain of social insurance, it could have been pursued more readily by other means. The government could simply have set up a "standard of need," an income target of minimal adequacy, graduated to allow for variations in family size, and provided to families or individuals the difference between their actual income and that standard. But we have never had such a general income support program. Indeed, although "negative income tax" programs modeled along these lines have been developed in great detail and proposed in varying forms by both conservatives and liberals over several decades, none has ever been adopted.[10]

Instead, as table 2.2 illustrates, we have many separate means-tested programs designed to secure the essentials of life and a "hand-up" to the needy. For all of these programs, recipients must be qualified not only by a lack of current income and resources but also by a complex set of family and personal characteristics that define special categories of the needy. These are the programs that have given rise to the "crazy quilt" image, a complicated, overlapping set of programs that negative income tax advocates have sought to replace. The question is whether the quilt is indeed a crazy one, and if not, what vision of public welfare unifies these apparently disparate efforts to assist the poor.

A simple altruistic sense that no American should fall below a certain level of subsistence is one motive for these programs. But they are also motivated by a desire to create opportunities for all Americans to become productive citizens. These programs not only provide a safety net against complete destitution; they are also programs of human capital investment. This is more obvious in programs of job training and job placement, rehabilitation services for the disabled, nutrition, and health care, but it is nonetheless true of the other major means-tested programs. Note, for example, how the Committee on Economic Security described its proposal for the federal grant-in-aid program that has become the current AFDC program:

[E]special attention must be given to the children deprived of a father's support usually designated [in the states] as the objects of mother's aid or mother's pensions laws, of whom there are now above 700,000 on relief lists. The very phrases "mother's aid" and "mother's pensions" place an emphasis equivalent to misconstruction of the intention of these laws. These are not primarily aids to mothers, but defense measures for children. They are designed to release from the wage earning role the person whose natural function is to give her children the physical and affectionate guardianship necessary not alone to keep them from falling into social misfortune, but more affirmatively to rear them into citizens capable of contributing to society.[11]

Although given to those whose current lack of resources is not only a recognized but an essential ingredient of their qualification, means-tested programs like AFDC were also meant to promote the development of economically independent adults.

This view is further supported by observing that although poor, able-bodied adults who have no children in their care make up the most impoverished of all socioeconomic groups in the United States, they have no national, means-tested programs, other than job training and placement combined with food stamps, available to alleviate their poverty. Having no children in their care and no obvious impediment to their own self-support, impoverished able-bodied adults can demand from the major programs of the American welfare state only a modicum of largely in-kind support while they prepare themselves for productive work.

A limited set of programs provide cash income and are based neither on insurance principles nor on a vision of investment in future capacity for self-support. Only for the disabled and the aged are there cash programs addressed strictly to the alleviation of poverty as evidenced by a means test. But these "residualist" programs are extremely small in relation to overall social welfare expenditures and have declined steadily in importance as social insurance has come to cover greater and greater percentages of the total population.

Indeed, means-tested programs were generally expected by the Committee on Economic Security to wither away as social insurance coverage became universally available. The New Deal's programs were not just oriented toward insurance and personal opportunity; they were actually hostile to the continuance of residualist "welfare" programs. But several things happened to prevent welfare's complete disappearance. First, social insurance never became universal. Ever since the abandonment of the work assurance part of the New Deal, the requirement of substantial attachment to the work force has always eliminated social insurance eligibility for some. Moreover, some basic programs of social insurance, such as universal medical coverage, have never been enacted. Second, the AFDC population shifted from widows with children, most of whom would have qualified for Social Security Survivors' Insurance, to families headed primarily by divorced or never married women. Finally, in the absence of any non–Social Security income from savings, workers' compensation, company pensions, or part-time work, some elderly and disabled Social Security beneficiaries are still poor enough to qualify for means-tested benefits. Nevertheless, these programs remain quite small and clearly residual.

Perhaps the most dramatic confirmation of the idea that insurance and opportunity define the basic parameters of the American welfare state is provided by the second great flowering of American social welfare programs—the so-called Great Society programs. Billed also as the "War on Poverty" and launched with great fanfare during the Johnson administration, they make up perhaps the least understood segment of the American welfare state. The misunderstanding is no doubt explicable. The Great Society initiatives were, in the public mind, predicated on the rediscovery of hunger and poverty during the 1960 presidential campaign. The situation was portrayed as a national embarrassment and the rhetoric of political mobilization suggested some straightforward attempt to relieve acute economic distress.

The simplest remedy, of course, would have been to send money. But this technique played virtually no part in any of the "War on Poverty" or "Great Society" programs. Instead, the programs created fell into our now familiar categories—programs of social insurance or programs to create economic opportunity. The major, indeed the only new, effort in the social insurance category was Medicare—a single program perhaps, but one that, while addressing a critical source of insecurity in old age has also become the second largest program in the whole of the American welfare state.

On the economic opportunity side of the ledger, the programs were legion, but their individual fiscal consequences were generally small. The Economic Opportunity Act of 1964 created a plethora of self-help, training, and professional assistance programs ranging from community action to Legal Services to Upward Bound to Head Start. Job training programs sprang up like mushrooms as a multitude of techniques were tried for different constituencies and subpopulations. Inadequate health care and child nutrition were attacked through Medicaid, community health centers, and a vastly expanded school lunch program. New federal funds were dedicated to basic education through Title I of the Education Act. Rural poverty was attacked through the creation of development authorities and commissions, urban poverty via model cities development programs.

Note that all of these programs have much to do with creating economic opportunity, or developing the capacities necessary to seize it, but nothing to do with income support. Indeed, the only initiative taken in an income support program during this period was to graft work and training requirements onto the AFDC program, along with a revision of income computation rules to benefit the working poor. In some sense, the impetus for both the New Deal and the Great Society programs was the fact of income poverty. But in neither period did American political institutions respond primarily by providing income. They provided instead economic opportunity and social insurance tied to the successful pursuit of such opportunities. In the Office of Economic Opportunity (OEO) programs, there was a slight "radical populist" spin, mostly in the rhetoric but also to a degree in the quickly dismantled "Community Action" component and the continuously embattled Legal Services program. But there again the emphasis was on organization for

42

self-help and the assertion of rights to opportunities already supposedly guaranteed by law.

This picture of the insurance-opportunity state is, to be sure, somewhat oversimplified. Programs of social insurance and economic opportunity *are* supported in part out of simple concern for the poor. And egalitarianism of a special sort, concern about racial injustice and its pervasive effect on the economic opportunities and positions of blacks, undergirded many efforts of the Kennedy-Johnson years. Social welfare programs are enormously complex amalgams of goals and techniques—a fact that we forget at our peril and that later chapters will be at pains to describe. Our concern here, however, is to depict the dominant unifying themes of American social welfare policy as they are embodied in America's social welfare programs.

We think it undeniable that those themes are both familiarly American and decidedly compatible with our dominant political ideology. The combination of economic opportunity and social insurance captures precisely the American political spirit. It harmonizes the Marlboro man with neighborly barn raising, rugged individualism with mutual support. The state's role here is to manage the background conditions of opportunity and to organize universal mutual support schemes. Its role is decidedly not, save in extreme last resorts, to provide unrestricted cash for the support of its poorer citizens. We have managed to preserve and further some aspect of every vision of social welfare purpose—behaviorist, residualist, social insurance, and radical populist—within an overarching institutional commitment to limited government and individual and local responsibility.

We should make clear, however, that although American commitments to economic opportunity and to mutual assistance are generally compatible with our broader political ideology, the programmatic articulation of these goals reflects ideological compromise, not transcendence of our differences. The frontier where conservative defenders of the principle of limited government do battle with liberal advocates of a more complete system of social insurance or of more generous assistance to the poor has always been sharply contested terrain. Moreover, the political strength of conservative ideological commitments and of conservative interests in the United States has been sufficient to hedge the American welfare state within narrower bounds than its guiding principles would seem to dictate. Some examples of what is *not* found in the complex of American social welfare programs illustrate these bounds.

First, note that a straightforward way to guarantee economic opportunity is to guarantee jobs. The government becomes either the employer of last resort or a direct contractor for labor-intensive projects in slack job markets. Both techniques were extensively used in the 1930s. The question to be answered then is why these programs were not maintained and expanded. Both were quite successful in putting Americans to work and in improving the physical infrastructure of the country. Both were clearly consistent with the work ethic and its social welfare analogue, the creation of economic opportunity.

The answer is in fact complex, but the simple part of the story is that conservative opposition defeated two major efforts to move the American welfare state in that direction. The first such episode came at the end of the Second World War in the congressional battle over the Employment Act of 1946, and the second came in the mid-1970s when a similar battle was fought over the Humphrey-Hawkins bill. Whatever the merits of the claims advanced by each side in those political battles, it is clear that the boundaries of the American welfare state are not elastic enough to encompass all means of extending economic opportunity to the poor. The lesson of all attempts to assure full employment in the United States has been that the logic of the work ethic trumps the logic of limited government only in emergencies, even if economic opportunity is thereby limited.[12]

The peculiarities and problems of our medical care programs provide another example of the boundaries that constrain the development of our insurance-opportunity state. The logic of social insurance surely extends to the cost of medical care. This logic has triumphed in every Western industrial democracy. Yet our public medical financing includes only the very poor, the elderly, the disabled, and veterans. Moreover, pursuing this partial public provision by simply agreeing to pay the charges of private providers creates truly extraordinary incentives for wasteful utilization of health care. The American system has managed to combine profligacy with inadequacy. Why such a bizarre system? Why not national health insurance on the Canadian or some other model? Again the answers are many and complex, featuring stories of the intransigent opposition of the medical profession and accounts of how our fragmented political institutions frustrate popular but contested demands. But the point to emphasize is that the profession's view has been politically powerful partly because it reflects ideological commitments and fears that extend well beyond the interests of one industry or profession.[13] This is another area where the American welfare state is bounded *within* the limits of its guiding ideology and constrained by its political architecture. As chapter 6 argues, we may get to national health insurance yet, but our ideas and institutions of limited government have thus far blocked the path to universal social insurance protection against the costs of illness and injury.

We should note also that the idea of limited government affects not just which programs we have, but also how they are organized. The fear of oppressive state power applies most forcefully in the American ideological context to the powers of the federal government. Limited government entails, therefore, not just a preference for private, nongovernment assistance to those in need, but also a preference for state or local, rather than federal, government provision. The federal government got into the act in a substantial way in the 1930s, in part because of the collapse of state and local fiscal capacity. And it is well-recognized that, even without a Depression-style collapse, there is a serious mismatch between the fiscal capacity of states and localities and modern conceptions of social welfare needs. Nevertheless, the disinclination to supplant state provision, at least state administration, persists. Many of the federal government's major commitments to social welfare are thus made in the form of grant or contract arrangements with the states or with localities. Virtually all cash assistance and economic opportunity programs for the poor take this form. Indeed, some ostensibly "federal" programs, for example the Social Security Disability Program, are entirely funded with federally collected dollars, yet administered almost entirely by state personnel.

As we shall see, federalism enormously complicates the politics of policy development and implementation in virtually every domain of social welfare policy except Social Security pensions. Those complications sink some programs, such as Community Action, and drastically limit the reach and efficacy of others. But the problem here is not just politics in some narrow sense of vested interests and bureaucratic turf squabbles. Battles over federalism form a key part of more generalized battles over social welfare policy in the United States.

When we say, therefore, that we believe Americans have demonstrated through their programs a political commitment to an insurance-opportunity state, we must always add that the state, at least the legitimate state, is a circumscribed one. The American insurance-opportunity state contains built-in limitations that dramatically distinguish its potential future elaboration from the almost limitless boundaries implied by the more general term "welfare state."

THE TRIUMPH OF DEMOCRACY?

To understand the American welfare state as an opportunity-insurance state having a special character and structure permits us to see its political coherence. The programs we have crafted fit the constrained political ideology just described. We have produced what reformers like to call a "crazy quilt" of programs that, even individually considered, contain compromises and "contradictions." But those are necessary for a polity that wants to affirm *both* self-reliance and mutual support, that believes *both* in the primacy of the market and in the necessity for collective action through government, that wants to rely on *both* national fiscal capacity and local political control.

Are we then claiming that American social welfare policy—that political sinkhole of failed ideas, obdurate bureaucracies, fraud and waste—is what the American people support? Indeed, if recent polling data are to be believed, this is close to the true story. Fay Cook and her colleagues at Northwestern University, for example, conducted an extensive survey of public attitudes concerning various American social welfare programs. The picture of public attitudes painted by an analysis of these survey results is a textured and complicated one. Nevertheless, there are generalities that are quite striking.[14]

The first is the very high level of support for existing programs. Respondents were asked, for example, whether they favored an increase, a decrease, or the maintenance of current levels of spending on Medicare, SSI (Supplemental Security Income), Social Security pensions, Medicaid, Unemployment Insurance, Aid to Families with Dependent Children, and Food Stamps. Respondents favored maintaining or increasing expenditures in all of these programs by overwhelming margins.

The listing of the programs in the preceding sentence is in descending order of public support, but support for all programs is very high. The percentage of respondents who wished either to increase or maintain expenditures for these programs ranged from a whopping 97.5 percent for Medicare to a still very healthy 75.6 percent for the Food Stamp Program. Moreover, with respect to the three programs viewed primarily as aiding the elderly—Medicare, SSI, and Social Security pensions—a majority support increasing expenditures. And although there are differences in levels of support based on the socioeconomic characteristics of respondents, the commonalities in attitude are much stronger than the differences.

The Cook survey also asked which groups in the society respondents were most willing to assist through government expenditures and probed the underlying attitudes that seemed to guide those preferences. Again, the picture that emerges is consistent and yet differentiated. There is greater support for food assistance for the aged and disabled than for either able-bodied adults or children. For education programs, respondents were more in favor of helping younger adults than the elderly. For coverage against catastrophic illness, they were more in favor of helping children than the elderly and more in favor of help to the elderly than to adults under 65.

The basic ideas of social insurance entitlement and human investment that inhabit our major welfare state programs seem to play substantial roles in this pattern of support. The Cook analysis puts the matter this way:

As with support for specific social welfare programs, members of the public differentiate in the reasons they give for helping particular recipient groups. When the elderly are preferred for a service, it is primarily because they are perceived to be the group with the least available other sources of help or because they are the group the public believes is entitled to help. On the other hand, when non-elderly adults are preferred, it is because the public believes the program can lead to independence and help the recipients be self-sufficient. When children are preferred, the reasons are future oriented—helping children is seen to be an investment in the future.[15]

We do not mean to suggest, of course, that citizen preferences are always translated into legislative action or that all legislative programs would receive even majority support if submitted to a referendum. Nor are we urging complete faith in polling results of any type. But this is not the place for extended discussion of survey methodology in the social sciences, nor of the bearing of the voluminous public choice literature on the democratic legitimacy of American social welfare legislation. Our claim here is sufficiently modest that we believe it defensible against virtually any version of public choice or methodological attack. The design of American social welfare programs is neither accidental nor incoherent. For nearly six decades American social welfare policies have elaborated a welfare state based on general principles of insurance and opportunity. These principles, and the programs that embody them, seem consistent both with America's historic political ideology and with the best evidence we have concerning current voter preferences. We have not somehow been led down the primrose path by shrewd policy elites or bumbled into a nightmare of fluffy ideals and contradictory policies.

Part of the climate of unease or dissatisfaction that surrounds America's social welfare programs may thus be nothing more than a failure of our political rhetoric to capture or create an image of what we in fact have wrought. It might help if we junked the term "welfare." Its associations in the public's mind are far removed from the actual content of the American welfare state. A substitute term such as "opportunity-insurance state" might be more accurate, but we are hardly sanguine that it will catch on.

THE NEED FOR A RATIONAL DISCOURSE

Nevertheless, we are far from convinced that our current national posture on social welfare issues is, or should be, one of self-congratulation. Although we find the apocalyptic critics of American social welfare policy to be singularly unpersuasive, we are not so naive as to believe that the status quo represents the best of all possible worlds. Neither global rejection of the American welfare state nor complacency regarding its problems is helpful. Although it is possible—just—that the welfare state we have constructed over the past fifty years is either perfectly suited or completely unsuited to our current and future needs, neither state of affairs seems likely. And although it is also possible—again just—that political realism about the likely path of American social policy would predict either complete stasis or massive reorganization, neither prediction is very plausible.

Yet, this commonsense vision is strangely absent from the general political debate about the American welfare state. Notice, for example, the place of Social Security policy in the presidential campaign of 1988. In the electoral contest itself, indeed, it had no place. Neither candidate would discuss it beyond a bland, if intense, commitment to complete maintenance of the status quo. Meanwhile, pundits abound who seem to relish attacking Social Security from almost every direction. Although their contradictory commentary makes it difficult to discern whether it is Social Security's impending deficits or impending surpluses that pose the greater threat to national economic health, their general message is clear. Something radical must be done to change Social Security pensions or our economy will soon be in ruins. In short, the talk to which most Americans are exposed concerning our largest social insurance program (the subject of chapter 5) sounds exactly like the extreme positions of success and failure that a moment's reflection suggests to be wildly improbable.

Take another example. We are constantly bombarded with claims that our welfare system has totally failed both to lift the poor out of poverty through income supports and to set them on the road to self-sufficiency through education, training, and

50

other social services. We have also recently been told by the Congress that it has completely overhauled the welfare system to make it measure up to our fundamental ideals. Welfare will now provide a hand up rather than a hand out; it will both eradicate poverty and cure dependency. Are Americans meant to believe this story of massive failure followed by total reform? We hope not. As we will demonstrate in chapter 4, the claims of both utter failure and fundamental reform are greatly exaggerated. Yet these exaggerations are the staple of our public fare.

To be sure, a mismatch between practical reality and political rhetoric is hardly unknown in other arenas of American public life. We live in a public world in which to be shrill is to be heard, in which both politicians and publicists continuously commit crimes against common sense. And yet we cannot escape the conclusion that, as it affects public understanding and discussion of the welfare state, this impoverished discourse is particularly unnecessary and pernicious.

It is unnecessary because over the past twenty years there has been much truly fine research on the problems and prospects of American social welfare policy.[16] More than that, there have been significant alterations in public policies, alterations that respond both to the changing socioeconomic conditions and to altered political demands. Within broad, but reasonable, parameters, we know what is happening, how and to what extent programs work, and how to alter them to make them better. Or, at least, "we know" if "we" means the specialist policy community that focuses full time on social welfare issues and that usually publishes its findings in professional journals and the little-read books of the academic presses. To read this literature is to experience neither the alarm nor the self-satisfaction that is engendered by attending to the more visible commentary.

The character of the public debate is pernicious because the absence of the specialists' knowledge from the visible public debate about social welfare policy undermines one of the most basic purposes of the American insurance-opportunity state itself, a purpose captured in the title of its largest program—to promote social security. We may know in our heart of hearts that neither intransigent defenders of the status quo nor apocalyptic critics are likely to be correct, but that hardly allays our anxiety in the face of an apparently empty realm of calm analysis and realistic alternatives. Polls that find continuing support for the welfare state also find rising concern about its stability and effects. The public is fearful both that the welfare state will not be there when they need it and that some part of what it is doing for some may be the wrong thing to do.

This book is dedicated to addressing these anxieties by exposing its readers to the ideas and findings of the professional literature that exists in this field beyond the realm of the popular media. It attempts to marshal some basic information about three major arenas of American social welfare provision—their development, current status, and likely future—and to present that information against the backdrop of the high rhetorical dudgeon that tends to populate contemporary public discussion.

We will return again and again to the principal critical claims of ungovernability, unaffordability, and undesirability. We believe these claims to be demonstrably false. And yet, to see why and how is also to see that there is a real and important agenda for reform that those concerns help identify. Entrenched interests *are* a problem, scarcity *is* ubiquitous, and it *is* hard to do good without also doing bad. What is missing from the critic's account is an understanding that American social welfare policy has always taken these concerns seriously. Missing from most defenses of current arrangements is the sense that it must continue to do so.

3

##

Crisis and the Welfare State

The welfare state is commonly portrayed as a child of crisis. Americans attribute their welfare state to the Great Depression and the New Deal response to massive economic insecurity. Germans tell a different crisis story, tracing the origins of their welfare state to conservative fears of socialism in the late nineteenth century. The British emphasize their nation's solidaristic response to the massive social dislocations caused by two world wars.

In each case the basic explanatory story is known to be partial, at best. The Depression may be a good explanation of the *origins* of the American welfare state, but it hardly tells us why our social welfare expenditures had their greatest growth forty years later. Conversely, wartime uncertainty and social solidarity may explain the major *growth* of the British welfare state, but not its origins. Nor can the need to contain socialism explain the maturing of the welfare state with the support of Socialists in twentieth-century Germany.

Yet, whatever their inadequacy, tales of welfare state origin and growth in the major Western democracies do have this in common—they feature social, political, or economic crises as the cause of welfare state activity. The development of social welfare policy is viewed as a response to national crises—as a device, or collection of devices, for reinstituting stability by responding to and ameliorating social, political, or economic insecurity.

Over the past decade and a half, however, the elite perception of the relationship between the welfare state and societal crisis has been changing. The emergence of stagflation as the central economic problem of the 1970s was associated with the propagation of the view that social welfare policy no longer functioned as a corrective for society's social, economic, and political troubles but was instead a primary cause of them. The continuance of low levels of growth, modest increases in productivity, and high unemployment rates throughout the 1980s could be attributed to the same causes.

The nature of the crisis allegedly brought on by the welfare state has been variously portrayed, but the charges leveled against it can be grouped under three headings. The first consists of claims that the welfare state is undesirable, particularly in its economic side effects. Proponents of this line of argument typically suggest that a return to the upward economic trajectory of the 1950s and 1960s requires a significant pruning, if not a dismantling, of the welfare state. Second, the welfare state is claimed to be unaffordable. Conservative commentators suggest that well-intentioned efforts to be generous in the distribution of benefits has led us to make commitments to broad strata of society that simply cannot be fulfilled without beggaring taxpayers.

The undesirability and unaffordability theses are combined by some left-wing critics into an even more pessimistic vision. Because the welfare state is viewed as necessary to maintain social peace in advanced capitalist societies, a growing conflict is foreseen between the claims of capital on society's resources and the need to maintain welfare state security. In short, the basic contradictions of capitalism have finally reached an acute phase. A capitalist political order no longer able to afford to bribe its victims with welfare state benefits must ultimately collapse. As Claus Offe has expressed this sentiment, "The contradiction is that while capitalism cannot coexist *with,* neither can it exist *without,* the welfare state."[1]

The third category of charges leveled at the welfare state involves claims of ungovernability. Even moderate observers who doubt the extreme claims of more radical critics frequently express dismay at the apparent rigidity of the welfare state. Economic troubles and uncertainties regularly implicate the welfare state in one way or another. Adjustments of some sort, perhaps of many sorts, are needed in welfare state institutions. But the entrenched interests surrounding welfare state entitlements render current arrangements politically sacrosanct. How can Western democracies adjust to their changed circumstances when special interests are so well positioned to block significant reforms? Our economy may not be threatened with imminent collapse according to this view, but its future will be a dreary one unless we somehow manage to break our political stalemate. Weighed down by a gradual accumulation of economic and social problems requiring significant adjustments in the welfare state, but forestalled from making needed changes by well-positioned special interests, we find our long-term prosperity in jeopardy. Lester Thurow, for example, sounds this theme in *The Zero-Sum Society.* "When there are economic gains to be allocated, our political process can allocate them. When there are large economic losses to be allocated, our political process is paralyzed. And with political paralysis comes economic paralysis."[2]

We believe that claims of social, political, and economic crisis attributable to the welfare state are either demonstrably false or wildly exaggerated. There is almost no evidence that high levels of social welfare spending have a depressing effect on an economy's rate of growth. Nor does the unaffordability thesis bear close scrutiny. Finally, the welfare state can be considered impervious to needed reform only if a dramatic and quick restructuring of its institutions is deemed essential. Incremental change and adjustment are possible, and experience in all Western democracies over the last decade and a half lends no support to the view that the welfare state is beyond political control. Economic, political, and social problems abound, but to blame them on the welfare state is misguided.

To acquit the welfare state of the economic crimes with which it has been charged is not, of course, to deny that it has shared in the troubles of our times. Since most modern industrial or post-industrial states *are* welfare states, state crises inevitably assume the form, at least in part, of crises in, or of, the welfare state itself. Our experience of stagflation may not be traceable *to* social welfare policy, but it certainly has created strain *for* social welfare programs. In periods of economic distress, claims on welfare state institutions rise disproportionately compared to the state's resource base. Politically difficult adjustments are required. A choice between benefit reductions and tax increases offers no joy to politicians. When the United States faced this choice in the late 1970s and early 1980s, a venomous distributional politics was unleashed. The dominant political tendency was conservative, but defenders of the welfare state were by no means silenced. Indeed, the public's continued support for the welfare state severely constrained conservative gains.

The dust from the battles fought over social welfare policy during that period now appears to be settling. The welfare state has suffered strain. It has been pared down at the edges. But the critics' agenda of wholesale cutbacks in entitlements generally has not been implemented. On the other hand, the confidence of the public, and of many elites, in the capacity of the welfare state to solve its problems has been badly eroded by the myths, misunderstanding, and misinformation disseminated by the system's critics. In addition, there is no clear sign that the fiscal constraints that have limited the growth of social welfare programs will ease in the near future. The lessening of international tensions may well produce some "peace dividend" for both the East and the West, but there are many domestic uses for these funds besides increased social welfare spending. In this political and economic atmosphere, new social welfare initiatives are likely to be modest. Social welfare programs are less beleaguered than they were in the early 1980s. The public has made it clear that it does not wish to roll back the clock, but the welfare state shows no signs of experiencing a renaissance either. Public confidence in the durability of welfare state institutions remains low.

This is unfortunate. A more positive view of our social welfare efforts is justified. The public has shown that it supports the programs constituting the American welfare state. It deserves to feel better about that support. There is no dearth of problems in the administration of individual programs; obvious gaps exist in the protection they afford; and practical achievements fall short of our aspirations. Still, claims that these programs actually harm the economy do not withstand close scrutiny. Nagging concerns that the welfare state may be responsible for sluggish economic growth, that it is unaffordable, and that its growth is beyond our control deserve to be dismissed.

THE (ECONOMICALLY) UNDESIRABLE WELFARE STATE

Before we begin, we want to make it clear that we are not here discussing the morally most controversial elements of the American welfare state, in particular, cash assistance to the able-bodied poor. "Welfare" is a perennial topic of controversy, but it is of very little significance to the fiscal difficulties of the modern welfare state. Because cash assistance programs for the able-bodied poor are so small, whatever "perverse incentives" they provide, they can have no significant impact on general economic productivity. We will document and elaborate these points in chapter 4. For now, we only want to avoid confusing the "crisis of the welfare state" with the "problems of welfare." The vast majority of welfare state expenditures are for social insurance programs that provide cash and in-kind assistance to persons who are not expected to work and who have earned their entitlement to welfare state support through prior contributions to social insurance. It is these large, politically popular social insurance programs that are at issue in debates over the economic effects of the welfare state.

The most common macroeconomic criticism leveled at the welfare state is that the relatively poor performance of all Western economies during the 1970s and 1980s is a consequence of overspending on social welfare programs. To assess this claim, we need to be clear what is meant by poor economic performance. In chapter 1 we reported data suggesting that the performance of the United States economy has deteriorated over the past decade and a half. These statistics focused on ways in which the economy's performance affected individual households—median family income, unemployment rates, and the rate of inflation. However, when claims are made that the aggregate effect of the welfare state is harmful to the economy, the concern expressed is usually more global—namely, that the overall rate of economic growth has suffered as a result of increases in social welfare spending.

Figure 3.1 portrays the growth of the United States economy from 1947 through 1989. As one would expect, given the performance data we reported in chapter 2, the period from 1947 through 1973 was one of more vigorous economic growth than the period since then. During the earlier period, GNP grew at an average annual rate of 3.7 percent, compared to only 2.4 percent for the more recent period.

Can this worsening economic performance be laid at the feet of the welfare state? In addressing that question, two features of the time series reported in figure 3.1 should be noted. The first is the key role played by recessions in reducing the economy's average growth rate during the latter period. The second

Figure 3.1   GNP Growth, 1947 to 1989[a] (1982 dollars, trillions, log scale)

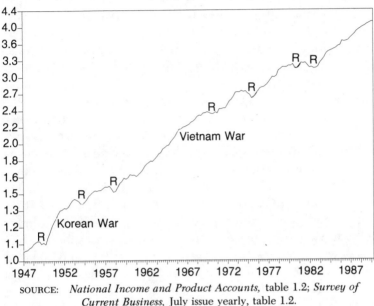

SOURCE: *National Income and Product Accounts,* table 1.2; *Survey of Current Business,* July issue yearly, table 1.2.
[a]R = Recession

is the important role played by two wartime mobilizations in boosting the economy's average rate of growth during the earlier period. In fact, if we disregard recessionary episodes in both periods, and also disregard the two episodes of very rapid growth associated with wartime mobilizations in the earlier period (seven quarters of growth at an average annual rate of 12.2 percent in 1950–51 and five quarters of growth at an average annual rate of 7.8 percent in 1965–66), the economy actually manifested very similar capacities for growth in the two periods. During quarters in which the economy was neither dragged down by recession nor artificially stimulated by wartime mobilization (76 quarters out of a total of 108 from 1947 through 1973, and 48 quarters out of a total of 64 from 1974 through 1989), growth rates averaged 4.2 percent both before and after 1973. Indeed, if we measured growth on a per capita basis during these quarters, the economy's expansionary capacity would appear higher in the later period.

It is true, of course, that market economies often post exceptionally high rates of growth after steep recessions, but the American economy's strong performance in expansionary periods since 1973 seems not to have been rooted in such a rebound. In fact, the average rate of growth in the five quarters following the end of a recession was greater in the pre-1973 period than it has been since. Nor can the economy's high average growth rate in post-1973 expansionary periods be attributed to particularly rapid growth during the 1980s. The economy's average growth rate from the end of the 1981–82 recession through 1989 was no greater than it was during the four and one-half-year expansion that followed the 1973–75 recession. In terms of average real growth rates, the supposedly disastrous late 1970s were just as good a period as the Reagan-Bush "boom" years. The current expansion has simply lasted longer.

The economy's average rate of growth *has* declined since 1973, but this trend has not been caused by a decline in growth rates across all phases of the business cycle. It is associated with deeper recessions and the absence of wartime stimuli in expansionary periods. Simplistic charges that social welfare spending has caused a general flagging in the economy's generative capacities are not supported by this record. Instead, the record suggests that events unrelated to the growth of the welfare state were at work. This is obviously true in explaining our avoidance of war, but it is also true of our business cycle experience over the past fifteen years.

Standard economic theory suggests that by helping to maintain consumption levels during an economic downturn, social welfare spending should actually lessen the severity of recessions, not deepen them. It is possible, of course, that there are indirect links between the growth of social welfare spending and the occurrence of deeper recessions, but in explaining the severity of our two major recessions since 1973, politics appear to have played a more decisive role. It is generally acknowledged that Oil Producing and Exporting Countries (OPEC) price increases and the Arab oil boycott both precipitated and deepened the 1974–75 recession. The Federal Reserve Board's determination to stamp out inflation with a tight money policy played a similar role in the back-to-back recessions of 1980–82. Growing social welfare expenditures, along with many other trends, certainly helped to shape the complex political and economic background that affected the working out of these events. But the claim that social welfare spending was at the root of these troubles involves a large measure of scapegoating.

The weakness of the claim that welfare state spending hurts economic growth is also demonstrated by comparative data. If growing social welfare expenditures depress growth rates, one would expect countries that spend more on social welfare programs to suffer from lower rates of economic growth. However, table 3.1, using data from the Organization for Economic Cooperation and Development (OECD), shows that over the period in which American economic growth has been recognized to be a problem, social welfare expenditures in Western industrial nations have had no consistent relationship to rates of economic growth. Neither the percentage of GNP spent on social welfare programs nor the rate of growth of social welfare expenditures has a consistent relationship with overall growth rates. The great variability of growth rates among both big social welfare spenders and small social welfare spenders suggests that other factors must play a decisive role in determining economic growth rates.

The lack of a clear correlation between social welfare expenditures and economic growth rates is not surprising if one considers the nature of these expenditures. Because social welfare

Table 3.1 Social Expenditures in OECD Countries 1960–1981[a]

Country	Social Expenditure as % of GDP		Annual Growth Rate of Real GDP (%)		Annual Growth Rate of Deflated Social Expenditure (%)		Decrease in Annual Growth Rate between 1960–75 and 1975–81	
	1960	1981	1960–75	1975–81	1960–75	1975–81	Real GDP	Deflated Social Expenditure
Canada	12.1%	21.5%	5.1%	3.3%	9.3%	3.1%	1.8%	6.2%
France	13.4[b]	29.5	5.0	2.8	7.3[b]	6.2	2.2	1.1
Germany	20.5	31.5	3.8	3.0	7.0	2.4	0.8	4.6
Italy	16.8	29.1	4.6	3.2	7.7	5.1	1.4	2.6
Japan	8.0	17.5	8.6	4.7	12.8	8.4	3.9	4.4
U.K.	13.9	23.7	2.6	1.0	5.9	1.8	1.6	4.1
U.S.	10.9	20.8	3.4	3.2	8.0	3.2	0.2	4.8
Average of above countries[c]	13.7	24.8	4.7	3.0	8.3	4.3	1.7	4.0
Australia	10.2	18.8	5.2	2.4	9.6	2.4	2.8	7.2
Austria	17.9	27.7	4.5	2.9	6.7	5.0	1.6	2.7

Table 3.1 (Continued)

Country	Social Expenditure as % of GDP		Annual Growth Rate of Real GDP (%)		Annual Growth Rate of Deflated Social Expenditure (%)		Decrease in Annual Growth Rate between 1960–75 and 1975–81	
	1960	1981	1960–75	1975–81	1960–75	1975–81	Real GDP	Deflated Social Expenditure
Belgium	17.4	37.6[d]	4.5	2.2[d]	9.3	7.9[d]	2.3	1.4
Denmark	—	33.3[e]	3.7	2.2	—	5.4[e]	1.5	—
Finland	15.4	25.9	4.5	2.9	7.5	4.8	1.6	(2.7)[f]
Greece	8.5	13.4[d]	6.8	3.5	8.4	9.4[d]	3.3	(1.0)[f]
Ireland	11.7	28.4	4.3	3.5	9.1	7.1	0.8	2.0
Netherlands	16.2	36.1	4.5	2.0	10.4	1.6	2.5	8.8
New Zealand	13.0	19.6	4.0	0.4	5.5	3.5	3.6	2.0
Norway	11.7	27.1	4.3	4.1	10.1	4.6	0.2	5.5
Sweden	15.4	33.4	4.0	1.0	7.9	4.7	3.0	3.2
Switzerland	7.7	14.9[e]	3.4	1.7	7.6	2.7[e]	1.7	4.9
OECD average[c]	13.1	25.6	4.6	2.6	8.4	4.8	1.9	3.8

SOURCE: *Social Expenditures, 1960–1981* (Paris: OECD, 1985), pp. 21 and 22, tables 1 and 2.
[a] Or latest year available. The definition of "Social Expenditures" is much broader in this table than it is in Table 3.2. For example, education expenditures are included only in this table.
[b] Excluding education
[c] Unweighted average
[d] 1980
[e] 1979
[f] Indicating an increase

spending is commonly measured by comparing it to GNP (or GDP, as we have done in table 3.1), it is easy to think of it as a drain on the economy's output, a wasteful reallocation of productive capacity from other uses. Viewed in this way, social welfare spending looks like it is absorbing a larger and larger share of total output, analogous to the allocation of a growing share of GNP to education, health care, or the production of armaments. It is therefore imagined that the money we spend providing social welfare benefits is unavailable for investment, and the large amounts involved seem like an enormous drag on our opportunities for economic growth.

What this view of social welfare spending misses is that such spending consists, for the most part, of transfer payments rather than direct purchases of the economy's output. When the government provides educational services or purchases military hardware, it does effectively commandeer productive resources that cannot then be used for other purposes (such as the accumulation of more physical capital). When the government issues a Social Security benefit check, however, it does not commandeer any productive resources. It merely transfers purchasing power from currently employed workers to Social Security beneficiaries. Transfer payments redistribute claims on the economy's output, but they do not directly determine how productive resources will be used. The public has the same aggregate purchasing power after the transfer is made as it did before. What is different is the relative size of individual claims on total output. The public as a whole is free to consume (or invest) just as much of GNP after the transfer as it was before.

Thus, the allegedly negative effect of social welfare spending on economic growth rates cannot stem from a direct withdrawal of productive resources from growth-inducing uses. A less direct chain of causation must be argued. There are, in fact, two basic arguments advanced by those who claim that social welfare spending harms the economy. The first is that transfer payments so cushion the shocks delivered by the economy that

64

individual adjustments to changed circumstances are sluggish and innovation is stifled. The second is that social welfare transfer payments encourage too much consumption, thereby depressing private saving and inhibiting investment in productive resources. Both of these arguments could have something to them. The question is how much.

We have already shown that there is no clear relationship between social welfare spending and economic growth rates. If the rigidities introduced into the economy by welfare state institutions really did have a harmful effect, we would expect to see such a relationship. The truth is evidently more complicated.

It may, in fact, be true that welfare state institutions do encourage some of the behavioral rigidities attributed to them by their critics. It is a long jump from that acknowledgment, however, to the conclusion that the *net* effect of those institutions is economically harmful. For example, virtually every serious investigation of Unemployment Insurance (UI) has found that the receipt of benefits lengthens the time it takes an unemployed worker to find a new job.[3] Standing alone, this effect harms economic performance because the return of jobless workers to productive employment is delayed. In other words, these workers become less flexible in their response to economic shocks.

However, UI has other effects that tend to improve the economy's performance. By automatically increasing government expenditures when the unemployment rate rises, and decreasing them when it falls, UI helps to flatten the business cycle. Also, by lessening the financial and psychological burden of involuntary unemployment on jobless workers, UI helps prevent the development of personal and family problems that both reduce worker productivity and impose significant social costs on society. Even the program's effect on job search behavior has positive as well as negative economic effects. An abbreviated job search in which an unemployed worker feels strong financial pressure to accept the first available job may not be economically optimal. Lengthier job searches may result in a better matching of unemployed workers to available jobs, thereby enhancing average worker productivity.

Like UI, all welfare state institutions have complex economic effects. Some are positive and some are negative. To demand of social welfare programs that they have no negative effects, even in the short run, would be silly. The sensible economic issue posed by welfare state critics is whether the *net* economic effect of welfare state provision is negative. The varied experience of countries with welfare states of differing degrees of generosity lends little support to the view that social welfare programs reduce an economy's productivity.

The suggestion that social welfare expenditures reduce savings also presents a superficially plausible story. Recipients of social welfare benefits generally have low incomes and cannot be expected to do much saving. If taxpayers did not have to pay for these benefits, they would find it easier to save. Moreover, if no one could count on government support payments to secure them from economic adversity, then everyone would have a strong motive to increase their savings.

Once again, reality is more complex than this simple picture suggests. Most of the research on the relationship between social welfare expenditure and private savings in the United States has looked at the effects of Social Security pensions on savings. As we explain in greater detail in chapter 5, the results of these inquiries are inconclusive. Researchers have found that Social Security taxes both increase and decrease private savings, as well as that they have no effect. After a careful review of the economic literature dealing with this issue, Henry Aaron and Lawrence Thompson conclude:

In general, social security may affect how much people save or work, but empirical analyses suggest that plausible variations in the program would produce small effects, if any. If policymakers conclude that saving or labor supply by older age cohorts should be increased, empirical research by economists on the effects of social security on such behavior suggests that the policymakers had better use other instruments if they want large effects.[4]

A look at cross-national data on social welfare expenditures and savings rates also suggests that there is no necessary relationship between the two. Comparatively high savings rates are as likely to coexist with comparatively high social expenditure rates as with comparatively modest social welfare expenditures (see table 3.2). The charge that the modern welfare state depresses savings is, to say the least, "not proved."

Moreover, given recent experience, that charge is peculiar on its face. The overall savings rate for an economy includes both public and private savings. Governments may, therefore, adjust net national savings through any number of policies that would stimulate either private or public savings—including the simple expedient of running surpluses in the public budget. Although it is quite problematic to claim that social welfare expenditure depresses private savings, we do know for sure that in the United States' budget the only accounts that were running in balance, or in moderate surplus, from 1975 forward were the social insurance accounts. The largest part of the American welfare state clearly was making a modest contribution to net national savings. And, of course, as the surpluses in the Social Security accounts grow from the present through the early decades of the twenty-first century, those accounts will make greater and greater contributions to net national savings.

It is, of course, also possible for the government to offset both public social insurance savings and private savings by running greater and greater deficits in other budget categories. But that is just to say that the overall savings rate is a function of overall government policy as well as the pattern, often unexplained and perhaps inexplicable, of private choices between consumption and savings. In sorting out these multiple effects, social

Table 3.2 Social Expenditures and Savings Rates in Major OECD Countries
1960–1985 (Percent of GDP)[a]

Country	Social Expenditures (Percent)				Savings Rates (Percent)			
	1960-67	1968-73	1974-79	1980-85	1960-67	1968-73	1974-79	1980-85
U.S.	5.4%	7.7%	10.3%	11.3%	9.8%	9.2%	7.7%	4.3%
Canada	6.5	8.2	9.9	11.4	9.5	11.1	11.6	8.8
Japan	4.1	4.8	8.4	10.8	20.6	24.6	20.2	17.4
U.K.	7.3	8.8	10.5	(NA)	10.0	11.3	6.6	5.9
France	15.5	17.2	21.0	25.4	15.1	16.0	12.0	7.2
Germany	12.4	13.2	16.7	16.8	18.2	16.9	11.5	8.8
Italy	11.1	12.0	15.4	18.5	16.2	15.2	12.1	8.8
Sweden	8.8	11.6	15.9	19.2	15.1	14.3	9.5	5.0

SOURCE: OECD, *Historical Statistics, 1960–1985*, p. 69, table 6.16, and p. 63, table 6.3.
[a]The definition of "Social Expenditures" is much narrower in this table than it is in Table 3.1. For example, education expenditures are included in Table 3.1 but not in this table.

welfare expenditures have no special relationship to the savings rate.

THE UNAFFORDABLE WELFARE STATE

There is some difficulty in understanding what is meant by the claim that social welfare expenditures are unaffordable. In one sense the idea is synonymous with the claim that social welfare spending limits economic growth: We can't afford the welfare state because it steadily shrinks the economic base from which it is financed. We have already explained why it is misguided to believe that social welfare expenditures are operating to limit economic growth either by their effects on the savings rate or their effects on work effort and labor mobility.

From another perspective, the "affordability" of the welfare state depends on our willingness to pay for it. In the ordinary private household, when we say we "can't afford" something, we normally mean that we don't have the cash or cannot finance it in a way that allows us to carry the capital costs of acquisition while maintaining other expenditures at desired levels. Translated to the public realm, this would be a claim that there are not sufficient tax revenues to finance current expenditures for social welfare programs and that the public is unwilling to pay sufficient taxes for their current support or for the debt retirement necessary to bring these accounts back into balance. As such, the claim is transparently false. The major American programs of social insurance are in current balance—indeed headed toward mammoth surpluses—and the public reports itself willing to pay more to maintain them at current levels. There is no deficit here of either fiscal capacity or fiscal will. Public willingness to support the smaller, noninsurance portions of the welfare state is not as strong as the support for social insurance, and its continued support is, therefore, not so certain should the economy worsen. But if we declared AFDC and Food Stamps "unaffordable" tomorrow and reduced their expenditures to zero, we would have erased only 10 percent of the overall budget deficit. These programs are simply too small to have much bearing on the affordability of the welfare state.

The unaffordability thesis can, however, be given a more sensible meaning. On this view, the claim is that the current level of social welfare expenditure, or the current rate of growth in social welfare expenditure, is not sustainable over the long run. We may not be currently bankrupt or unwilling to support our social welfare habit, but the time is coming—perhaps rapidly—when both of those situations will be upon us. The call then is to recognize, not a current crisis, but one that is developing inexorably for the future. In order to see the plausibility of this thesis, we need put together only three trends.

The first trend is the flattening of growth in median family income shown in figure 1.1. Since the oil shock of 1973, the growth of family income that we had come to expect, based on nearly thirty years of postwar experience, failed to materialize. We have not really gotten poorer, but we expected to get richer. As a consequence, we feel that many things are becoming unaffordable. Indeed, some items of consumption crucial to our sense of well being have become less affordable. This is particularly true of housing. The sustained inflation and high interest rates of the period since 1973 have had a dramatic effect on the affordability of home ownership. In 1973, the typical 30-year-old male could carry the mortgage on a median priced home by expending only 21 percent of his gross earnings. By 1984, this percentage had climbed to 44 percent. The flat trajectory of the growth of income, along with a more than doubling of the percentage of income spent on housing, goes a long way toward explaining the population's growing sense that its available discretionary income is shrinking. And a sense of constrained circumstances translates quite easily into resistance to the government's demand for support through taxation. We might then believe that the citizenry, whatever they say when polled about their willingness to pay more for social welfare programs, is in fact close to the limit of its tolerance for taxation. That certainly was the belief of the successful presidential candidates during the 1980s.

Next look at the trend of government payments to individuals as a percentage of gross national product (see figure 3.2). Whereas median family income has been flat from 1973 to the present, the trend line for the major social welfare programs slants dramatically upward. And, because most of those payments go to families with incomes below the median, it seems clear that the burden on middle-income taxpayers to support social welfare programs has increased dramatically.

Now, for the third trend, consider the demographics of dependency. We already know that a major share of American social welfare expenditures goes to pensions and medical care for the aged. Because those programs are funded largely on a "pay as you go" basis—that is, the contributions of current workers support those who are now retired—the burden on current workers is a function of the ratio of employed to retired persons. The more workers per retiree, the less each worker must contribute to provide the retiree with an adequate income. That ratio in turn is primarily a function of birth rates (although the percentage of working-age individuals actually in the labor force is also influential). Look then at figure 3.3. In that figure, the baby boom of the late 1940s through the early 1960s is dramatically evident. Almost all of these baby boomers are now in the work force, many of them in their prime earning years. By the second decade of the next century, the first part of the baby boom will reach retirement age. Meanwhile, the labor force will consist increasingly of workers from the low birth-rate years that began in the 1970s. As time goes on, the ratio of workers to retirees will decline. By the middle decades

Figure 3.2   Government Payments to Individuals, 1949 to 1984
(Percent of GNP)

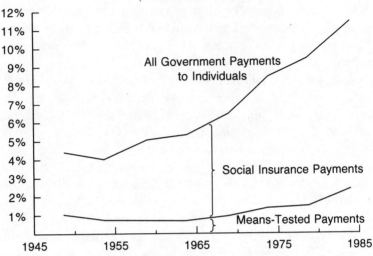

SOURCE: F. Levy, *Dollars and Dreams*, Russell Sage Foundation (1987),
p. 167, figure 8.4. Reproduced with permission.

of the next century, the prospect is that for every two workers contributing to Social Security there will be one retired worker drawing benefits.

The converging trends of flat real incomes, rising commitments of GNP to social welfare expenditure, and increasing numbers of persons eligible for social welfare payments suggest real trouble. Indeed, these trends are already being billed as creating a looming war between generations. The last five years has seen a spate of articles, in both elite and popular journals, decrying the American welfare state's propensity to cosset the wealthy aged while burdening the impoverished young. New "educational" groups have begun to spring up under such labels as "Americans for Intergenerational Equity." The title of an article that appeared in *Forbes* magazine perhaps captures the

Figure 3.3   The United States Birthrate, 1910 to 1986
(Births per 1,000 women ages 15–44)

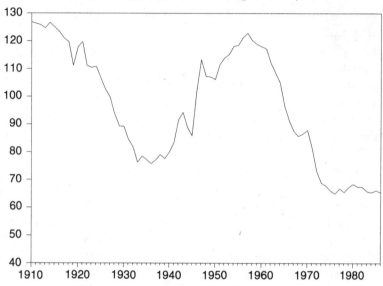

SOURCE: *Historical Statistics of the U.S.*, Series B, 5–10, p. 49. National
Center for Health Statistics, *Vital & Health Statistics,* "Trends and
Variations in First Births to Older Women, 1970–1986," table 4, p. 17,
June 1989 (Series 21, No. 47).

tone of the emerging commentary; it is called quite simply,
"Consuming Our Children."[5]

We have no desire to rebut the notion that the extrapolation
of the three trend lines we have been discussing into the in-
definite future would produce some form of economic, social,
and political upheaval. There surely would be a real crisis in the
welfare state. The question is why anyone should believe that
those trends will continue as they have over the past decade
and a half. Fertility rates, for example, have a chronic, if somewhat mysterious, tendency to change over time, sometimes

73

dramatically. There is, indeed, evidence of a modest resurgence in American fertility rates in recent years. The U.S. fertility rate bottomed out at 1.74 in 1976. Since then it has fluctuated but with a slight upward trend. In 1986, the last year for which data are available, it was 1.86. And even if fertility rates remain low, perhaps *because* of their low levels, median income may turn up as each worker is supported by greater and greater amounts of physical capital. In addition, concentration on the aged misrepresents the real trend line of dependency that will shape demands on the welfare state.

The number of aged persons dependent on each potential worker is, indeed, growing, but the number of children needing such support is shrinking even more. When the young and old are combined, the total "dependency ratio"—the percent of the population not expected to be available for productive work—is declining. In 2040, fifty years from now, the dependency ratio still will be lower than it was in 1960.[6]

In short, the unaffordability thesis is, in general, either confused, incorrect, or rigid in its extrapolation of relatively recent experience into the distant future. For present purposes, however, let us not question the inexorable decline in the worker/retiree ratio or the static quality of real median income. On those assumptions, the only trend line that seems clearly controllable through public policy is the trend of social welfare payments. But, say the fearful, these increases seem to have a life of their own. Or, put more concretely, because the old are so numerous and politicians so feckless, we are unlikely to be able to bring the welfare state under control. From this perspective, the claim that the welfare state will become unaffordable merges into the belief that it is ungovernable.

THE UNGOVERNABLE WELFARE STATE

Those who believe that the welfare state has become ungovernable, that the trend of social welfare expenditure is fixed in an upward trajectory hardly susceptible to downward adjustment, point to some obvious difficulties in social welfare policy-making in the United States. Both the major political parties and the internal institutions of the Congress (committees, party caucuses, and other leadership institutions) have been declining in power for several decades. Along with presidents, representatives and senators now tend to appeal directly to the voters. Each congressional office operates as a largely independent political unit. But freedom from party and leadership discipline is a mixed blessing. These independent political entrepreneurs find that their day-to-day activity is carried out increasingly under the watchful eyes of powerful interest groups. Some of the most numerous and, therefore, most powerful of these groups are those who support the continuation and enlargement of welfare state expenditures, particularly for the aged. If the tales of the journalists are to be believed, congressional representatives live in particular fear of the displeasure of the American Association of Retired Persons. To be soft on support for Social Security and medical care for the aged, including proposals for their expansion, is to court political disaster.

The behavior of recent presidential aspirants lends credence to the journalistic accounts. Perhaps the only headway that Walter Mondale made against the Reagan juggernaut in 1984 was to create doubts about Reagan's commitment to the preservation of Social Security. Those doubts were so damaging that Reagan became, almost overnight, a rigid defender of the status quo. Similar attempts to portray the opponent as a possible "raider" of the Social Security Trust Fund punctuated the Bush-Dukakis presidential contest and elicited from the candidates the same sorts of reflexive rigidity. To hear the candidates speak was to believe that adjustments in the welfare state, particularly those aspects dealing with the aged, were to be ruled firmly off the public policy agenda for the foreseeable future.

The question is what hope we might have that the candidates will govern better than they campaign. After all, the idea that some of the most massive expenditures in the public budget are to be immune from adjustment, in the light either of changing circumstances or changing preferences, borders on lunacy. Are we now in a situation in which politicians must both make and keep promises that prevent necessary adjustments in social welfare spending?

That we are seems extremely doubtful. The history of Social Security policy-making, for example, has been a history of incremental adjustment. Since 1935 the amendment process has been almost continuous in the Congress. To be sure, over much of this period the agenda of change was a politically palatable agenda—the expansion of benefits. But this has not been true since the mid-1970s. Since that time, the politics of Social Security inside the Congress has been largely a politics of containment, if not retrenchment. Substantial changes designed to control runaway expenditures in the disability insurance program were adopted in 1980. Major adjustments in both the taxation and benefits sides of old-age pensions were accomplished in 1983, following close upon Congress's 1981 and 1982 cuts in Medicare spending and its less than adequate pension adjustments in 1977. Although the Medicare adjustments of the early 1980s have clearly been inadequate to ensure long-term solvency, the changes in disability and pension policy have, by all reasonable estimates, established fiscal balance in the pension and disability programs for the foreseeable future. Indeed, as we discuss in greater detail in chapter 5, current controversy surrounding pensions largely concerns what to do about the projected and enormous surpluses that will build up in the pension funds during the next three decades.

The political processes leading to these adjustments were

hardly smooth or painless, and there clearly have been unhappy lags between recognition and solution of social insurance difficulties. Yet, if one looks at the growth rate of American social expenditures as a whole in the critical years of altered economic expectations, the adjustments in spending began almost immediately after the oil shocks of 1973 revealed that we were in for a period of economic troubles. Social expenditures from 1960 through 1975 grew at a real rate of 8 percent. From 1975 through 1981, by contrast, the growth rate was only 3.2 percent. Moreover, these reductions brought social spending growth almost exactly into alignment with the reduced growth in our gross national product. Although social spending was growing in the period 1960 to 1965 at a rate nearly 2½ times as fast as GNP, over the period 1975 to 1981 social expenditures and GNP grew at exactly the same rate. Our institutions governing social welfare responded to a real economic crisis both quickly and dramatically.

Similar tales of economic strain followed by adjustments in the rate of growth of social welfare spending characterize the behavior of other countries during the same period. Look again at table 3.1, which shows the changes that occurred in overall economic growth rates and in social expenditures growth rates in OECD countries before and after the economic troubles of the 1970s took hold.

These data demonstrate that the worst scenario of those who argued that uncontrollable growth in social welfare spending would bankrupt Western democracies was being falsified at the very time it was being popularized.[7] Average economic growth rates in OECD countries declined from 4.6 percent in the 1960–75 period to 2.6 percent in the 1975–81 period. This 43 percent decline in overall growth rates was exactly matched by a 43 percent decline in the average growth rate of social spending in these countries—from 8.4 percent in the 1960–75 period to 4.8 percent in the 1975–81 period.

The response to slower growth in the seven largest OECD

countries was even more dramatic. Their average rate of gross domestic product (GDP) growth declined less than the overall OECD average, from 4.7 percent in the 1960–75 period to 3.0 percent in the 1975–81 period. This 36 percent decline in overall growth rates accompanied a 48 percent decline in the average growth rate of social spending—from 8.3 percent in the early period to 4.3 percent in the latter period. Among this latter group of countries, the American response was the most extreme of all. Our average GDP growth rate declined only marginally between the two periods, but we reduced the rate of growth in our social programs by an enormous 60 percent.

When economic expectations changed, the major spending programs of the welfare state did not continue to grow as if uncontrolled by political authorities. Expansion did not continue automatically in the midst of fiscal strain. Everywhere, review and restraint took place. This restraint was all the more remarkable since deteriorating economic conditions meant that claims on welfare state institutions were increasing. If anything, the United States overreacted to the onset of stagflation, stalling the development of needed social welfare programs.

That we have adjusted to changing economic conditions in the past, even the recent past, does not guarantee that we will have the political will or foresight to make necessary adjustments in the future. But neither does this history justify dire predictions of impending collapse, bankruptcy, or intergenerational warfare. There are surely challenges to be faced, but that is not even a rough equivalent of the declaration that the welfare state is currently or foreseeably in crisis.

THE CHALLENGES AHEAD

There is no reason to believe that the current size or character of the American welfare state is a serious impediment to economic growth, threatens us with imminent public bankruptcy, or makes adjustment and "steering" of social policy and expenditure impossible. For all the talk of "crisis" in the welfare state, there is precious little evidence to bolster that claim. The institutions of the welfare state have not reflected—either in their programmatic actions or by their inability to adjust—the sense of critical disjuncture that hostile intellectuals have managed, with the help of some politicians, to popularize.

But rejecting these alarmist assessments does not imply that the welfare state faces no troubles or anxieties, or that adjustments in appropriate directions will be made easily in the years ahead. The problems and prospects of particular areas of welfare state policy-making are the subject matter of most of the chapters that follow. For now we should attend only to some structural issues that are a common backdrop against which those specific policy debates will be played out.

The first structural feature that should be recognized is that substantial pieces of the American welfare state are now mature. The large programs of social expenditure—retirement pensions, disability pensions, survivors' pensions, and medical care for the aged—are programs in which the vast majority of Americans participate, and they are funded at levels that permit benefit payments of reasonable adequacy. In these areas, the welfare state has become the status quo, shaping our understanding of our current economic situations and our expectations for the future. This limits the possibilities and prospects for radical change. Reprivatization of these social risks is not on any realist's political agenda. Nor is a substantial expansion in the generosity of these major social insurance programs. Across-the-board increases in social welfare spending would require increases in either taxes or public sector deficits, which the public is in no mood to sanction. Thus, welfare state adjustments will almost certainly be at the margins. Large increases in expenditures are conceivable only in small programs.

When social welfare expenditures, broadly defined, make up nearly half of the federal budget[8], those expenditures cannot grow at rates exceeding whatever bonus is provided by GNP growth generally without enormously constraining the opportunities for all other expenditures.[9] When the welfare state represents 10 percent of national public expenditure, it can grow five times as fast as GNP while leaving half the GNP growth bonus for other public purposes. When the welfare state represents one-half of national public expenditure, a growth rate five times as fast as GNP not only eats up all the GNP surplus, it requires an increased level of taxation simply to maintain social welfare spending growth. Competition for public fiscal resources is unlikely to allow this to occur.

Second, the incremental adjustments that are feasible may be made in appropriate directions only with difficulty. Most would agree, although we seldom focus on the fact, that American social insurance provision for the aged has been a very substantial success. That very success, however, has created constituencies that make adjustment, even marginal adjustment, a laborious political undertaking. And the strength of these constituencies creates the ever-present threat of new and unsustainable expansions of programs whenever surpluses appear. Honoring interest-group demands for changes in an expansionary direction is made easier by the high level of support for social insurance programs among the general public and by the focusing of political responsibility for these programs on the federal government.

By contrast, programs for the nonaged are often morally controversial, lack support by well-organized interest groups, and involve substantial participation by the states. Children don't vote and the poor are unorganized. Even if these constituencies had surrogate political actors who made strong demands for their support, those actors would face the organizational difficulties of diffuse state responsibility and the economic reality of limited state fiscal capacity. As a consequence, it is hardly surprising that the adjustments in the American welfare state during the late 1970s and the 1980s have cut much more substantially into programs for the nonaged than for the aged. There is a looming, indeed present, imbalance in our social welfare provision that is extremely difficult to address.

As we shall detail in chapter 6, redressing imbalances in health care provision will also be difficult. Resistance by health providers and insurers, by the business community generally, and by state and local policymakers has until now defeated rationalization of American medicine and its financing. Part of the basic social insurance package, identified in the Committee on Economic Security's Report in 1935 and available in every other Western democracy, is missing from the American welfare state. In health, public policies and public needs seem badly out of synch. And, as we shall also see, the cost of this frustrating stalemate has been not only continued insecurity but rampant medical inflation as well.

To the extent that there is a sharp challenge to the American welfare state, therefore, we believe it is a challenge of appropriate governance. The problem is not that the welfare state is ungovernable; rather it is that the various aspects of social welfare policy are differentially governed. The welfare state can both expand and contract, but it has a tendency to expand more and to contract less in some areas than in others. This results from structural features of contemporary American government that are constant across multiple episodes of incremental policy revision. The result may be a balance among various aspects of welfare state provision that, as a general policy matter, is neither justified nor justifiable. This challenge is, of course, not peculiar to social welfare policy. It affects all of American public policy-making. But it is a problem with which welfare state provision must grapple nonetheless.

4

Welfare, Poverty, and the Welfare State

Over the past several years we have repeatedly quizzed our colleagues, students, and other nonspecialist acquaintances about their understanding of American social welfare policy. We have been particularly interested in their conception of the place "welfare" occupies in the "welfare state" and in their view of the relationship between American welfare efforts and the incidence of poverty. We have heard expressed repeatedly the same ideas—a collection of beliefs that reflect, in distilled form, the reporting of both the daily press and standard journals of news and commentary concerning welfare in America. On our view, there exists something like a set of standard beliefs among well-educated adults concerning welfare, poverty, and the welfare state.

The standard belief goes something like this: First, by "welfare," most people mean cash assistance for needy families provided by the Aid to Families with Dependent Children program (AFDC). Second, "welfare," so defined, is viewed as a substantial and growing component of American social welfare expenditures. Third, AFDC in particular, and means-tested programs in general, are viewed as the government's primary weapons in combating poverty. Finally, there is, if not a conviction, at least a concern that these massive expenditures have failed to turn the tide in the war against poverty. Many people adopt the even more pessimistic view that welfare actually has contributed to the incidence of poverty. "Welfare," in short, is seen as having failed in its essential goals.

This conclusion, what might be called the failure thesis, undergirds what some regard as the new consensus on welfare, a consensus heralded by the legislative leaders who produced our most recent federal welfare reform, the Family Support Act of 1988.[1] In the vision that they, and others, have marketed to the American people, welfare policy is now being taken in a revolutionary new direction. Entitlements to cash income are to be replaced by entitlements to job training and job placement, and cash relief is to be conditional on work effort. Under this new regime, welfare's creation of dependents, its deleterious effects on family stability, and its tendency to reinforce a cycle of poverty will be a thing of the past.

There is a straightforward problem with these standard beliefs concerning welfare's place in the American welfare state. Many, indeed most, of them are false. The consequences of this misunderstanding, moreover, are not benign. Not only do we risk misapprehending what we should want to do about our welfare programs, but we simultaneously deny ourselves the possibility of recognizing our past successes and of developing sensible expectations about the likely prospects of programmatic reforms. The result is a sense of anxiety, if not dismay, about past efforts combined with extravagant hope for new initiatives. A more accurate picture would emphasize the partial, but sometimes quite dramatic, successes of the welfare state's overall assault on poverty while highlighting the serious problems that existing programs, including the welfare reforms of 1988, address only obliquely. Let us examine one by one the familiar myths, misapprehensions, and half-truths that undergird the standard view in an attempt to replace them with what we take to be the true state of welfare in the American welfare state.

THE SIZE, GROWTH, AND CHARACTER OF "WELFARE"

As data in table 4.1 reveal, the belief that the American welfare state has grown dramatically over the past two decades is surely correct. Total federal spending has risen spectacularly since the 1960s, whether measured in terms of total dollars spent or as a percentage of either total federal spending or gross national product.[2] But "welfare" is not "the welfare state."[3] Indeed, once we begin to dig into the numbers, we discover that social welfare spending and welfare spending have followed radically different paths.

First, take a look at spending for AFDC, the program that most people equate with welfare, detailed in table 4.2. The facts are startling, given the common view that welfare expenditures constitute a substantial and growing component of the American welfare state.[4] In real terms, AFDC spending was lower in 1987 than it was in 1971. As a percentage of total federal social

Table 4.1   Federal Social Welfare Expenditures,
1960–1987

(Billions of 1988 Dollars)

Year	Total	Percent	
		Federal Spending	*GNP*
1960	$ 99.5	28.1%	4.9%
1965	141.2	32.6	5.6
1970	235.3	40.1	7.8
1975	367.9	52.0	11.0
1980	434.6	54.3	11.3
1985	496.8	48.6	11.5
1987	519.8	50.4	11.3

SOURCE: *Social Security Bulletin* 52 (Nov. 1989): 20, table 1.

Table 4.2   AFDC Benefit Payments, 1965–1987

Year	Total Benefit Payments[a] (1988 Dollars, Billions)	Total Payments as % of GNP	Federal Share as % of Total Federal Social Welfare Spending[b]	Federal Share as % of Total Federal Spending[b]
1965	$ 6.2	0.24%	*	*
1966	6.8	0.25	*	*
1967	8.0	0.29	*	*
1968	9.7	0.33	*	*
1969	9.6	0.38	*	*
1970	14.8	0.50	11.2%	4.4%
1971	18.1	0.59	12.3	5.4
1972	19.5	0.60	12.4	5.7
1973	19.2	0.56	11.1	5.5
1974	19.0	0.56	9.9	5.0
1975	20.2	0.60	8.6	4.3
1976	21.1	0.60	7.9	4.2
1977	20.7	0.55	7.3	3.9
1978	19.4	0.49	6.4	3.4
1979	18.1	0.45	5.7	3.0
1980	17.9	0.47	5.2	2.7
1981	16.8	0.43	4.6	2.4
1982	15.8	0.41	4.2	2.1
1983	16.4	0.42	4.0	2.0
1984	16.5	0.39	3.9	1.9
1985	16.7	0.38	3.7	1.8
1986	17.3	0.38	3.7	1.8
1987	17.1	0.36	3.6	1.7

SOURCES: Total benefit payments from *Social Security Bulletin*, Annual Statistical Supplement, 1988, table 5.3. Federal social welfare spending from *SSB*, Nov. 89, p. 30, table 1. Federal AFDC expenditures from *Background Material and Data on Programs within the Jurisdiction of the Committee on Ways and Means* (Washington, D.C.: GPO, 1989), p. 556, table 18.

[a] Calendar year; includes federal, state, and local funds.

[b] Fiscal year; includes administrative expenditures.

*No data available

welfare expenditures, of total federal outlays, and of GNP, it has also shrunk. Nor is this shrinkage trivial. In relation to total spending by the federal government, AFDC has been cut to less than a third of its former relative size. At less than 4 percent of total federal social welfare spending, AFDC is fiscally an insubstantial part of the American welfare state. At less than two-fifths of one percent of GNP, this program's contribution, if any, to our current fiscal strain is vanishingly small.

Why are popular impressions of the size of welfare programs so wide of the mark? There are several answers to this question, and all are important for understanding the American welfare state and the quite different public assistance system for low-income persons that we actually have constructed. There is a tendency to equate "welfare" with AFDC, to equate both with the "welfare state," and to regard the latter as synonymous with "antipoverty" programs. As a comparison of the welfare state's growth with AFDC's relative decline makes clear, some of these equivalencies are wildly wrongheaded. Welfare is a minuscule fraction of the American welfare state.

It would, indeed, be astonishing to find cash assistance to poor families dominating the expenditures of the American welfare state. Our welfare state, remember, is not primarily directed at the alleviation of poverty. Its principal purpose is to insure workers and their families against common risks. Assistance for destitute individuals and families is only grudgingly provided unless it is perceived as a "hand up" to self-improvement and productive employment. Because AFDC is not an insurance program and has a problematic relationship to the goal of encouraging self-sufficiency, we should not expect it to be more than a marginal element of a welfare state having the ideological underpinnings we have described.

The Growth and Decline of AFDC. But the public is not composed of fools. Instead of being totally out of touch with reality, common presumptions regarding the growth and fiscal significance of AFDC simply may be out of date. In the first seven years of the series reported in table 4.2, expenditures for AFDC more than tripled, and they increased almost as much when compared to GNP. There clearly *was* a growth period in AFDC. Had that growth rate continued, AFDC would now be a very substantial component of the American welfare state.

Prevailing ideas about welfare may have been formed in the go-go years of the late 1960s and early 1970s, when "poverty wars" and "welfare reform" dominated the discussion of social policy. Since the American welfare state as a whole continued to grow after this period, the public may have assumed that "welfare" continued to grow along with it. This explanation of current standard beliefs as being simply anachronistic leads, of course, to a further puzzle. Why did welfare grow so fast for a short period and then stop? Piecing together that puzzle has something important to tell us about the dynamics of American welfare policy.

In explaining the period of AFDC's rapid growth, a good guess might be to describe AFDC's salad years as simply a part of the flood of federal dollars that funded Lyndon Johnson's Great Society. A good guess, but slightly off the mark. In fact, in its orgy of enactments and appropriations directed at a wide range of social ills, the Great Society congresses of the Johnson era made no substantial changes in the AFDC program.

The so-called Great Society programs, particularly Community Action and Legal Services, did, however, have an effect on welfare. They created a cadre of federally financed advocates for the poor who set about to improve the lot of their clientele. These advocates quickly discovered many, many poor families who were eligible for Aid to Families with Dependent Children but were not receiving it. In part, this situation resulted from lack of information on the part of those who were putatively eligible. It also resulted from the continuous resistance of many

87

state and local welfare offices to the full implementation of the AFDC program. As a consequence, Community Action case-workers, Legal Services attorneys, and others mounted an effective campaign to qualify the previously unqualified for AFDC. Particularly in the hands of the lawyers, a program that had long been viewed as a form of public gratuity was rapidly recharacterized as one entailing "welfare rights."[5]

Nor should we imagine that the story of this period is simply one of the victories of welfare rights advocates over recalcitrant welfare administrators. During the same time that the welfare rights champions were mounting their campaigns, their contemporaries, whose liberal social consciences also had been honed in the civil rights struggles of the 1950s and 1960s, were finding their way into the administration of public assistance and into electoral politics, both as voters and as candidates. At least some state legislatures responded to the political ethic of the War on Poverty and the vision of the Great Society by increasing levels of support under the AFDC program. They thereby qualified for aid substantial numbers of the working poor whose incomes had previously disqualified them. And, of course, these increased payments went to existing recipients as well. Meanwhile, the liberalization of eligibility practices in state and local welfare offices, both as a result of legal changes and as a result of changes in the social perspectives of their personnel, qualified and raised the support levels of thousands more. In this atmosphere, persons who were eligible for AFDC were also more likely to view their entitlement as a right they could pursue with dignity rather than as a form of charity to be shunned. Many of these changes in policy, practice, and attitude were small. But because they were virtually all in the same direction, together they added billions of dollars of expenditure to the AFDC program.[6]

Why, then, did AFDC stop growing in the early 1970s? First, of course, some of the factors that fueled the program's growth had natural limits. The population of eligible persons was not growing rapidly. The enrollment of those previously eligible but not yet attached to the program could not fuel growth forever. Moreover, after 1973 we entered a world beset by stagflation and strained government resources. This might have been less important if AFDC were a wholly federal program. But it is not; nearly half of its monies come from state treasuries. A jump in federal AFDC payments would be noticeable but much less painful for the federal government to absorb because of its greater fiscal resources. That same increase at the state level, where revenue sources are more limited and budgets must be balanced, has a far more dramatic political impact. With tax revenues stagnating and AFDC payments rising, state legislators balked at appropriating more money for the program. Because there was no federally mandated scale of payments, states were under no legal obligation to raise payment levels. And in the face of significant inflation, holding payments virtually constant over the next decade meant that AFDC would experience the relative decline shown in table 4.2.

Yet there is more to the story than this. AFDC is a state-federal program whose payment levels are determined primarily by states' willingness to pay. But welfare need not be structured in this way. Cash payments to the poor might have continued to grow substantially if the recharacterization of welfare benefits as a substantive right had really taken hold. If welfare had been transformed into a federally mandated right, entitling single mothers to levels of public support sufficient to reduce poverty significantly, then the political retrenchment of state legislatures would have been forestalled. The War on Poverty could, after all, have been fought with federally mandated transfer payments to the poor.

But this federal, cash-assistance War on Poverty never materialized. Concerted efforts, in both the Nixon and Carter administrations, failed to enact welfare reform packages that looked very much like a negative income tax. In part these efforts failed because of a peculiar alliance between southern legislators who thought the reform proposals too generous and welfare rights champions who thought them too stingy. Nor should one exclude from the reasons for failure the difficulty of coming to any agreement concerning the financing of a substitute for AFDC that would be acceptable both to most of the states and to the federal government.[7]

In a more profound sense, however, we believe that these efforts failed because they were not pursuing a political ideal that was particularly attractive to the mass of Americans. Establishing income support as a basic right of citizenship is not for most Americans a high priority. To many it seems absurd. American cash assistance to the poor has never been about rights. It has been about the alleviation of suffering, largely without strings attached for those not expected to be in the work force, but with plenty of strings attached for those who are expected to be self-supporting. From that perspective the small, personalized, state-federal AFDC program looks much better than a negative income tax, even a heavily disguised one. AFDC was thus left a state-federal program. That fiscal and administrative arrangement not only limited the growth of the program in the 1970s and 1980s; it will also be an important determinant of how the program operates in the 1990s. That is an issue to which we will return later in discussing the 1988 Family Support Act.

Welfare Beyond AFDC. There is thus a grain of truth in popular misconceptions about the growth of welfare. Moreover, that grain might have another added to it if we recognize that "welfare" should really include more than AFDC. Perhaps there has been substantial growth in payments to, or on behalf of, the poor, but they simply do not show up in the AFDC budget. After all, we have already noted the great outpouring of legislation from the Congress that created, among other things, the Community Action and the Legal Services programs. Surely the broader War on Poverty spent *some* money on the poor.

Indeed it did. During the Great Society years Congress created two noncash or "in-kind" programs to aid the poor that now cost the federal government substantially more than the AFDC program. One of these was Medicaid, which finances medical care for certain categories of poor people. The other was the Food Stamp program, which gives subsidized vouchers to low-income persons for the purchase of food. A glance at figure 4.1 will show that, unlike AFDC, federal Food Stamp expenditures continued to grow until the early 1980s and Medicaid expenditures are still growing.

In addition to Medicaid and Food Stamps, the Congress in 1974 federalized three federal-state grant-in-aid programs for special categories of the poor—the blind, the aged, and the disabled. These three programs were combined into what is now called the Supplementary Security Income program (SSI). As figure 4.2 shows, that program, unrestrained by state fiscal malnutrition and containing an automatic benefit adjustment to compensate for inflation, has also grown significantly from its inception to the present. In fact, the federal government now spends more on SSI than it does on AFDC, though combined federal, state, and local expenditures are still greater for AFDC.

Nor do these programs exhaust the activities that have been undertaken on behalf of the poor through means-tested programs. Look again at table 2.2. Targeted help is provided through a variety of programs in addition to Medicaid, AFDC, Food Stamps, and SSI. Indeed, funding for over seventy smaller programs is also included in table 2.2. They include relatively well-known programs such as the Job Corps, Head Start, Guaranteed Student Loans (now called Stafford Loans), subsidies for low-rent public housing, and the School Lunch Program. But many of the programs are not well known—health centers for migrant farmworkers, nutrition programs for the elderly, rural housing repair loans, the foster grandparents program, social

Figure 4.1   Federal Food Stamp and Medicaid Expenditures, 1965–1988 (1988 dollars, billions)

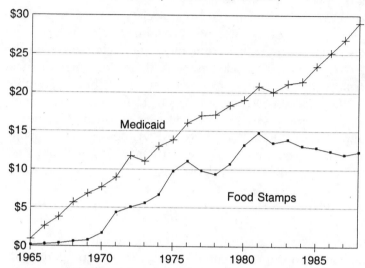

SOURCE: U.S. Library of Congress, Congressional Research Office, *1990 Budget Perspectives: Federal Spending for the Human Resource Programs,* 1965–1988 (Feb. 2, 1989), p. 79, table 4.3.

services for refugees, and a host of others. If *all* these efforts are what is meant by "welfare," then perhaps there has been a substantial increase in government assistance for the poor.

A look at table 4.3 reveals this, indeed, to be the case. In constant dollars, means-tested program expenditures for low-income persons increased by almost three and a half times between 1968 and 1988. The public is thus not completely bonkers in believing that over the past two decades we have made some substantial increases in our welfare efforts, provided welfare is understood to include all programs for low-income persons.

Figure 4.2 Supplemental Security Income Expenditures, 1975–1988 (1988 dollars, billions)

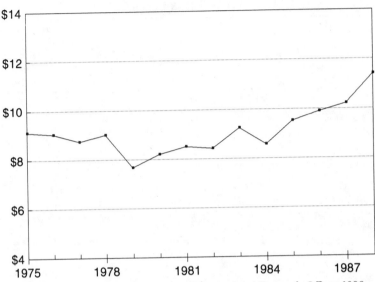

SOURCE: U.S. Library of Congress, Congressional Research Office, *1990 Budget Perspectives: Federal Spending for the Human Resource Programs,* 1965–1988 (Feb. 2, 1989), p. 79, table 4.3.

Four things, however, must be kept firmly in mind in order not to jump to erroneous conclusions about the state of welfare spending in the American welfare state. First, most of this growth, like the growth in AFDC, was in the earlier part of the period. From 1968 to 1973 means-tested spending increased at the whopping average rate of 12.9 percent a year. Over the next five years it grew at an average rate of 9.3 percent. However, from 1978 to 1983 the average growth rate of means-tested spending by all levels of government was less than 1 percent. Indeed, from 1981 to 1982 such spending actually

Table 4.3   Spending for Means-Tested Benefits
1968–1988, Selected Fiscal Years
(Billions of 1988 Dollars)

FY	Federal Spending	State & Local Spending	Total[a]	Growth Rate[b]	Total as % of GNP	Federal as % of Total Federal Spending
1968	$ 36.6	$ 15.1	$ 51.7	(NA)	1.9%	6.4%
1973	68.9	25.9	94.8	12.9%	2.9	10.9
1978	112.4	35.4	147.9	9.3	3.9	14.0
1983	112.6	40.6	153.3	0.7	3.9	11.7
1988	125.6	47.5	173.0	2.4	3.6	11.8

SOURCE: U.S. Library of Congress, Congressional Research Service, *Cash and Non-Cash Benefits for Persons with Limited Income: Eligibility Rules, Recipient and Expenditure Data,* FY 1986–88 (24 Oct. 1989), pp. 9–12.
[a] Total means-tested spending by all levels of government.
[b] Average annual growth rate of total means-tested spending by all levels of government over preceding five-year period.

declined by 3.1 percent because of a 5.2 percent cutback in federal expenditures. If medical and educational assistance is ignored, the reduction in federal means-tested spending was 11.5 percent that year.[8] This was an especially significant reduction, since it occurred amid a steep recessionary contraction, when means-tested spending usually increases. Since 1983, total means-tested spending has grown more slowly than GNP while accounting for a relatively constant share of total federal spending. The overall welfare expenditure story is thus one of initial growth followed by partial retrenchment, the same pattern we found in chapter 3 for American welfare state spending in general.

Second, even when welfare is broadly defined to include all means-tested spending, it makes up less than 30 percent of total welfare state spending by all levels of government. The American welfare state is mostly social insurance, not "welfare" or even "antipoverty" programs.

Third, the "welfare" part of the welfare state is a source of fiscal strain largely because of its state-federal organization. Outlays for welfare are too small to be of major importance to federal deficit reduction—the issue that has so dominated national political discourse for the past decade. Federal AFDC expenditures totaled only $10.8 billion in 1988. The federal budget deficit, excluding the help provided by surplus Social Security tax collections, was $244 billion. Even when we count as welfare all means-tested aid to low-income persons (including medical care, food aid, housing benefits, educational assistance, job training, and energy assistance in addition to cash aid), the total bill comes to only about half the deficit total. Moreover, the history of federal and state expenditures reveals that welfare programs are obviously a controllable part of the welfare state. This is a tap that can be turned off, as well as on, down, as well as up. Neither unaffordability nor ungovernability even remotely characterizes welfare expenditures.

Finally, notice that the broader set of programs directed at low-income persons, our expanded conception of welfare, contains very little that is morally controversial to most Americans. The "welfare" of phrases like "the welfare mess" and the "cycle of poverty," is a welfare of cash payments to working-age adults. And that, as regards national programs of public assistance, can only mean the fiscally trivial program of Aid to Families with Dependent Children.

Fiscal triviality is not necessarily a ground, of course, for public contentment with AFDC. Indeed, because that program now supports children, a majority of whom bear the stigma of having been born out of wedlock, and because our collective beliefs about whether the caretaker adults of small children, particularly mothers, should be in the work force have changed substantially since 1935, AFDC is certain to be controversial. We should not, however, make the mistake of thinking that our most politically problematic program is either a substantial drain on the public purse or that it is in any way emblematic of the American welfare state. That is to give AFDC a fiscal role that is wildly disproportionate to its actual size and a symbolic role that is profoundly mistaken concerning the program's relationship to the core ideals that undergird America's commitments to its more consequential social welfare programs.

WELFARE AND POVERTY REDUCTION

So much for the place of welfare in welfare state fiscal arrangements. What about the relationship between welfare, the welfare state, and poverty? The conventional wisdom, of course, is that welfare and the welfare state have failed to solve the problem of poverty. But the stories about the dynamics of this failure are radically different. In one version failure is attributable to lack of effort. We never fought the cash War on Poverty that might have been ushered in by the family-assistance plans of either the Nixon or Carter administrations. And the great growth of the welfare state, in social insurance payments, has not been targeted at the poor. A competitive version views our antipoverty expenditures as sufficient to cure income poverty if giving money to the poor could actually cure poverty. On this view, the persistence of poverty is powerful evidence of the pernicious tendency of welfare to produce, rather than alleviate, dependency. Once again, however, the conventional wisdom is badly mistaken.

What Has Happened to Poverty?   Changes in the incidence of poverty in the United States are sensitive to what is measured, how, and over what time period. The most basic measure that we will use is the "official" poverty estimate reported by the Census Bureau's Current Population Survey (CPS). That estimate focuses on absolute levels of self-reported, annual cash income. There are many reasons to view this poverty estimate skeptically.[9] Nevertheless, the census numbers are the most widely used by the press, commentators, and policymakers, and they have been compiled systematically over a considerable period of time. The CPS figures thus provide a reasonable picture of trends even if the absolute levels of poverty reported are contestable and contested.

First, the numbers for the past three decades simply belie the claim of failure. The CPS reports that the incidence of poverty fell from 22.2 percent in 1960 to 13.5 percent in 1988, a decline of 39 percent. We *have* made progress in reducing poverty over the past 30 years. This reduction might even be described as substantial. To be sure, this progress is attributable to rising average income levels as well as to government transfer programs, but the latter have had an important effect. In 1987, the nation's overall poverty rate would have been 20.6 percent instead of 13.5 percent were it not for these transfers.[10] Moreover, the decline has been greater than these figures suggest, because the CPS data do not take into consideration the increasing importance of in-kind benefits in boosting the real income of poor households. If the value of food and housing benefits were counted, contemporary poverty rates would be 1.5 percentage points below the reported figures.[11]

To be sure, although these data belie the general critique that the United States has made no progress in eradicating poverty, all such progress cannot be attributed to social welfare efforts. Moreover, that even 10 percent of the population of the richest nation on earth should be poor is certainly cause for concern. And, finally, a closer look at the overall trend line described by the CPS takes a good bit of the bloom off the rosy picture of declining poverty rates that we have painted.

Figure 1.3 illustrates two disturbing facts about the decline in poverty rates that has occurred over the past several decades. First, almost all of the progress we reported occurred before

1970. Second, we were not doing as well against poverty in 1984 as we were in the 1970s. After a period of steady progress in reducing poverty rates, we seem to have bogged down, even gone backward. Thus, the public's gloomy view of poverty trends over the past two decades is not unfounded. We need to know why our antipoverty efforts have stalled, and how this experience reflects on the success or failure of the American welfare state.

It is also possible that the public is unimpressed with our longer-term progress against poverty because it has heard something about how much we have paid to achieve it. After all, the poverty gap, the difference between the incomes of the poor before taxes or transfer payments and the amount necessary to raise all families to the poverty floor in any given year, is far less than the amounts spent each year on social welfare programs. In 1987, for example, the poverty gap was about $124 billion, while welfare state expenditures totaled more than four and a half times that amount.[12] Spending for means-tested programs alone, those presumably targeted at the poor, totaled close to $159 billion.[13] Is this not evidence of, if not a failed, at least a spectacularly inefficient welfare state? We will approach these issues in reverse order.

Antipoverty Efficiency. Two things need to be understood under this heading. One is straightforward, if occasionally rather technical: Poverty reduction is a very imprecise measure of the efficiency of even our means-tested, cash-assistance programs. The other is an apparent paradox: Poverty reduction has been accomplished largely through programs that do not target the poor.

The efficiency of a program is, broadly speaking, a measure of its capacity to conserve resources while accomplishing its purposes. An antipoverty program that closes 10 percent of the poverty gap at a cost of $15 billion is more efficient than a program that has the same effect at a cost of $20 billion. It is also more efficient than a program that spends $15 billion but closes only 5 percent of the poverty gap. So far so good.

Now, which programs of the American welfare state are explicitly designed to close the poverty gap? Answer: None. Such a program is, of course, imaginable. It would be a negative income tax that used the poverty line as its standard of need. To the extent that the income of a family or an individual fell below the poverty line, a payment would be made sufficient to bring them up to the poverty floor, but no higher. No one already above the poverty line would receive anything. Unless such a program had extremely high administrative expenses it should be very efficient at achieving its clear, and apparently single, objective—closing the poverty gap.

But, as we previously explained, Congress has consistently refused to adopt such a forthright program of poverty reduction. The programs that make up the American welfare state are quite different. Social insurance payments are based, not on demonstrated lack of income, but on prior contributions and the occurrence of a defined risk—death, disability, retirement, or medical expense. Means-tested programs providing cash assistance are largely directed toward groups that have experienced similar risks but are either not covered or not adequately covered by contributory social insurance programs (the aged, blind, and disabled poor, and children who have either lost or never had the support of one or both of their parents). Means-tested programs providing in-kind assistance (Food Stamps, medical care, shelter, job training, and the like) are primarily intended to contribute to the recipients' capacity for independent living and eventual self-support. Viewed as an assault on poverty defined in terms of a lack of current cash income, these programs are quite inefficient—they are over- and undergenerous, as well as over- and underinclusive. But as we have repeatedly stressed, direct poverty reduction is but one purpose of the American welfare state and not the sole purpose of any of its programs. Any program will appear inefficient if its efficiency is judged in relation to purposes different from those it is actually designed to serve.

To worry about the efficiency of the American welfare state from the perspective of an interest in eliminating poverty is thus really to worry about the *purposes* of our current welfare state and its programmatic expression. If there is a failure here, it is a failure of aims, not of execution. There is no evidence that a significant portion of welfare state expenditures is going to the wrong people or for the wrong purposes or at excessive administrative expense. Perhaps we should have a welfare state directed primarily at the elimination of the current income poverty of all Americans. That we do not now have one signals, not that our welfare state is inefficiently administered, but that it is pursuing different goals.

The idea that a more efficient antipoverty welfare state requires an alteration in our current programs and their goals is, of course, not a new one. It was one of the guiding principles of prior unsuccessful efforts to enact something like a negative income tax. And it animates some current suggestions for redirecting social insurance payments to the truly needy. In both cases, however, reformers talk primarily about better targeting of payments to achieve more efficient antipoverty effects. What is missing from their talk is an appreciation for the diverse goals that actually animate the American welfare state—a failure that inevitably leads to frustration and ineffective policy prescription.

To see this more clearly, let us recast our inquiry into antipoverty "efficiency" in terms of antipoverty "effectiveness." The revised question is not, "Which programs have the greatest percentage of their dollars targeted on the poor?" but, "Which programs eliminate the largest percentage of poverty?" The answer is the paradoxical one that we mentioned earlier: cash social insurance payments, the programs that most clearly are *not* directed at the poor, are the most effective at reducing poverty.

As table 4.4 shows, the difference between the effectiveness of social insurance and means-tested cash transfers in lifting people out of poverty is quite staggering—700 percent in 1985. In that same year, social insurance payments were nearly three times as effective as means-tested cash and in-kind programs combined. Nor is this differential effectiveness limited to the aged poor. Although social insurance, particularly Social Security retirement pensions, clearly has its greatest antipoverty

Table 4.4 Antipoverty Effectiveness of Major Income Transfers, Selected Years 1967–1985

Year	Cash Social Insurance	Cash Means-Tested	All Cash Transfers	In-Kind Transfers	All Transfers
Percentage of All Poor Persons Removed from Poverty by Various Transfers					
1967	22.7%	4.7%	27.3%	(NA)[a]	(NA)[a]
1979	33.2	6.3	39.6	10.2%	49.8%
1985	30.3	4.2	34.5	7.1	41.6
Percentage of All Elderly Persons Removed from Poverty by Various Transfers					
1967	44.9%	6.3%	51.3%	NA	NA
1979	66.9	13.9	83.6	NA	NA
1985	71.3	14.0	85.3	NA	NA
Percentage of All Nonelderly Persons Removed from Poverty by Various Transfers					
1967	11.0%	4.7%	15.7%	NA	NA
1979	18.1	9.0	27.1	NA	NA
1985	15.4	4.1	19.5	NA	NA

SOURCE: Isabel Sawhill, "Poverty in the U.S.: Why Is It So Persistent?" *Journal of Economic Literature* 26 (1988):1100, table 5.

[a] Fully comparable data not available, but estimates suggest that the antipoverty effectiveness of all transfers was probably only half a percentage point greater than the antipoverty effectiveness of cash transfers alone in the mid-1960s.

impact on the aged, social insurance payments to the disabled and to the survivors of deceased workers eliminate nearly four times as much poverty among the nonaged poor as do means-tested cash benefits. The conclusion is thus inescapable: In the United States, social insurance has been a dramatically more effective antipoverty strategy than has welfare. Or, to put it in terms of our paradox, efficiency is ineffective.

The reasons for this paradox are not hard to find. Although their poverty is not the occasion for a social insurance transfer, many who receive social insurance payments would otherwise be poor. Because Social Security now covers over 90 percent of the population and pays substantial benefits, it has large effects. Perhaps more important, because social insurance has overwhelming popular support, it is much more resilient politically in times of fiscal strain. The last dozen years have seen considerable retrenchment in means-tested programs, while social insurance cutbacks during that time have been extremely modest. Returning to table 4.4, notice that whereas means-tested cash benefits lost a third of their overall antipoverty effectiveness in the period 1979–85, social insurance lost only 9 percent of its antipoverty effectiveness. And while the power of social insurance to lift the non-aged poor out of poverty declined by 15 percent in that period, cash welfare payments lost 54 percent of their antipoverty efficacy.

Notice also that the most resilient and most effective programs have been those for the aged. This is true even of the means-tested programs. The most significant antipoverty success story is Social Security pensions, which now prevent destitution among 71 percent of the aged. The growth of welfare state transfers between 1967 and 1985 reduced the poverty rate for elderly individuals by almost 12 percentage points, and most of this progress was attributable to the growth of social insurance benefits rather than means-tested programs.[14] The elderly have thus been transformed from the age group most likely to suffer from poverty into the age group least likely to be poor. Recalling Fay Cook's polling data from chapter 2, which revealed that Americans are substantially more willing to provide cash transfers to the aged than to any other group, this is truly an instance of Congress putting the public's money exactly where the public wants it spent.

A Brief Recapitulation. We now know a fair amount about the state of welfare and poverty in the American welfare state. Cash assistance to the poor has never been a large part of our welfare state and is literally dwarfed by social insurance expenditures. This pattern of expenditure fits our preferences for pooling common risks and the creation of opportunity as the primary functions of the welfare state. The American public may care about the elimination of poverty, but it is not keen on addressing income poverty through the simple expedient of cash transfers to the poor. Fortunately, however, our large and growing welfare state, particularly its social insurance component, does prevent much poverty. As the American welfare state has grown over the last three decades, the rate of poverty has declined by nearly 40 percent.

Yet there are some disturbing aspects to what we have wrought. First, we have made no progress against poverty since the mid-1970s, and, judged by legislative actions, our willingness to support means-tested benefits for the poor has eroded. Have we reached some critical juncture in our capacity and willingness to aid the poor—a juncture that looks rather like a cul de sac? Second, the efficiency/efficacy paradox poses a serious threat to further progress. There are limits both to the extension of social insurance coverage and to increases in social insurance benefits. Our most effective antipoverty programs are not only our most expensive, they also omit from their largesse the worst off of our citizenry, those without steady employment. Third, many believe that instead of looking for ways to expand social insurance as an antipoverty tool, we should be concentrating our attention on reducing the federal budget deficit.

We have not yet considered the most fundamental challenge to the vision of welfare, poverty, and the welfare state that we have been developing. That challenge comes from those who believe that any notion of solving the poverty problem by expanding either means-tested *or* social insurance transfers is self-defeating—that such efforts will increase real poverty rather than alleviate it. Indeed, the claim is that our current and past efforts have increased rather than lessened poverty.

We will have more to say toward the end of this chapter about the prospects for further poverty reduction through either welfare or social insurance reforms. We will have much more to say about social insurance and the federal budget deficit in chapter 5. We turn now to the question of whether the welfare state's successes in reducing poverty have actually been an illusion.

WELFARE AND DEPENDENCY

Why did progress against poverty stagnate in the early 1970s? Why did the incidence of poverty actually grow in the early 1980s? Why did both of these results occur while overall welfare state expenditures were steadily increasing? Charles Murray provided a widely publicized answer to these questions that captured the imaginations of many in his 1984 book, appropriately entitled, *Losing Ground.*[15] The welfare state must spend more and more to do less and less, said Murray, because it actually aggravates the problem it is ostensibly designed to solve. Welfare generates rather than reduces dependency.

The World According to Murray. From this perspective the substantial success story we have been telling is instead a story of failure. We should be looking not at how many are poor *after* welfare state transfers, but how many are poor *before* those payments are made. The welfare state should be viewed as a success only if the pretransfer or "latent" poor are declining. The numbers show that this is not the case. The latent poor are in fact increasing. Why? Murray claims that it is because the welfare state encourages dependency. It gives people money and other support for taking up positions in society for which transfers are available. We are now simply spending more and more to support the dependents that we have created and continue to create. The only solution is to stop making the payments.

Murray buttressed his case with a wealth of statistics and appealing stories. *Losing Ground* is forcefully, sometimes brilliantly, written by an author who evinces deep concern for the plight of the poor. It encountered an audience similarly concerned and also increasingly anxious about government spending, economic decline, and the increasingly visible problems of homelessness and the so-called underclass. For these reasons Murray's analysis has been widely believed and highly influential even when sharply criticized. It has become a part of the conventional wisdom; indeed, it is so much a part of conventional thinking that to talk about welfare and dependency after *Losing Ground* is for many to talk in the terms of that particular analysis. Yet, we do not think it unfair to characterize Murray's arguments as composed largely of misunderstanding and misdiagnosis. Almost nothing Murray says about the effects of welfare or welfare state policies on the poor is believed by serious students of the subject.[16]

A basic failing in Murray's argument is one we have already encountered. His approach is enormously overgeneral. Does he really mean that income transfers and other supports are causing people to get old, to become blind or disabled, to need medical care? Not really. In fact, of the welfare state's major support programs, Murray is really only concerned with "welfare," principally AFDC. And since we know that the major growth areas of the welfare state have been elsewhere, the image that Murray conjures up of massive expenditures on antipoverty efforts to no, or to detrimental, effect is just that—image, not reality. Taking "welfare" in its broadest sense of means-tested programs, he could be talking about somewhere between 14 percent and 23 percent of welfare state expenditures. Yet, throughout *Losing Ground* he often seems to be talking about much, much more.

To put the point slightly differently, Murray's idea of increasing "latent poverty" or "dependency" suffers from a seriously misleading lack of focus. "Dependency" sounds like a bad thing, but that is because we tend to associate it with particular subgroups of the "latent poor," those whom we believe should be supporting themselves. Does Murray really think, for example, that the very substantial reduction of poverty among the aged over the past twenty-five years has been a bad thing? Would he argue that Social Security pensions should be viewed as having created a group of "dependents" who represent a serious social welfare policy failure? Again, clearly not. He has simply used a technical term, "latent poverty," interchangeably with a pejorative label, "dependency," to justify a massive and unnecessary sense of disquiet about our social welfare arrangements.

What then is Murray really concerned about? The answer is straightforward: young, unemployed males and young, unmarried females with illegitimate children, especially among blacks. Now let us get one thing straight at the outset. We agree with Murray that these are people who deserve our concern. Youth unemployment, illegitimacy, and the formation of female-headed households are indeed serious problems. They are highly associated with poverty, and they are particularly concentrated in poor black communities. The question, however, is what the relationship is between these problems and welfare.

Charles Murray's response to this question is put in terms of a hypothetical couple named Harold and Phyllis. They are young, poorly educated, unmarried, and prospective parents. As the blessed event looms, the question for Harold and Phyllis is what to do about getting married and getting jobs. As of about 1960, Murray's view is that Harold and Phyllis are likely to marry and one or both of them will get jobs. As of about 1970, the same situation would produce abandonment of Phyllis by Harold, with Phyllis going on welfare when the baby arrives. In Murray's account, the difference in these choices is the result of changes in welfare eligibility and payments during the decade of the 1960s.

That account is superficially plausible. According to Murray, Phyllis could have gotten about $70 a week from AFDC in 1960 (measured in 1984 dollars). This is hardly enough for her and the baby to live on alone, and she cannot live with Harold because the welfare office checks up on living arrangements. A "man in the house" would render her ineligible for AFDC payments. Hence, if Phyllis does not marry Harold, she has to live with her parents or put her baby up for adoption. Married to Harold, on the other hand, they might both get minimum wage jobs (making about $125.00 a week each), provided some arrangement can be made about the baby. And even if only Harold worked, at the minimum wage they would be about as well off as Phyllis would be alone and on welfare.

The situation confronting Harold and Phyllis, according to Murray, has changed dramatically by 1970. The eligibility rules and payment levels for welfare are substantially different. The Supreme Court has struck down the man-in-the-house rule. Hence, Phyllis could accept AFDC and live with Harold, thereby combining AFDC with his earnings. Moreover, if Harold does not acknowledge the child as his own, his earnings won't count against Phyllis's AFDC standard of need. AFDC payments in 1970 are roughly equivalent to what Harold could make at a minimum-wage job. The obvious solution for Harold and Phyllis is to remain unmarried, live together, and collect AFDC. Indeed, even if Harold does not find steady work, the couple is better off living on Phyllis's AFDC than they would have been on Harold's minimum-wage job in 1960.

On the basis of the Harold and Phyllis story, Murray invites us to imagine tens of thousands of Harolds and Phyllises making individual decisions in response to the new incentives provided by the welfare system. When added together, those decisions are meant to explain the rise in illegitimacy, AFDC participation, and labor force nonparticipation that we have observed from the 1970s to the present.

Harold and Phyllis create an extremely powerful image of the dynamics of welfare dependency. We have taught *Losing Ground* to scores of students and, if they remember anything from reading the book, it is the Harold and Phyllis story. Moreover, Murray's story convinces many that he is on to something important about the relationship between welfare, dependency, and social pathology.

Yet, as knowledgeable reviewers have pointed out time and again, the Harold and Phyllis tale is wrong. It misrepresents the facts of welfare eligibility and it is internally inconsistent. Moreover, broader measures of the relationship between welfare payments, illegitimacy, and work effort demonstrate that the dynamic suggested for Harold and Phyllis simply does not operate for the tens of thousands who might be in roughly their circumstances.

Consider first the facts of welfare payments and eligibility. Murray's story uses the state of Pennsylvania as the hypothetical home of Harold and Phyllis. Pennsylvania was a high benefits state in 1960 and an even higher benefit state in 1970 in comparison with the whole of the United States. If average AFDC benefit payments for the country as a whole were used, the numbers would not add up in the way Murray makes them add up in Pennsylvania. Overgeneralization is again at work in Murray's analysis. Overreading is also evident. The Supreme Court's decision concerning the man-in-the-house rule decided only that states could not presume that any man with whom an

AFDC mother had a continuing liaison was providing support to her and her children equal to the whole of that man's earnings. It did not prohibit AFDC offices from inquiring into the actual contributions of persons who were resident in an AFDC household or prevent any state from making it an offense punishable by criminal penalty to misrepresent the family's actual income on an AFDC application. Harold and Phyllis could live as Murray suggests, but they would have to perjure themselves in response, not just to one, but to multiple inquiries concerning their current income and resources. They would have to deny Harold's paternity consistently and to assert constantly that he provided no support to Phyllis or the baby, although sharing their household.

Perhaps more important from an economic standpoint, the decisions that Murray has Harold and Phyllis make in 1970 make no sense. If Harold is not going to work, then there is no reason for Phyllis to let him live with her and the baby and share their meager AFDC check. This is as true in 1970 as it was in 1960. Likewise, both in 1960 and in 1970, a Harold who is supporting himself at a minimum-wage job is worse off economically if he includes in his household an AFDC child and mother. Either marrying Phyllis or living with her will lower his standard of living.

In short, what the Harolds and Phyllises of the world do about their awkward situation will be determined by a host of factors other than changes in welfare payments: what their parents think, what their friends think, how they feel about adoption or abortion, how Harold feels about joining the army or working at McDonald's, how Phyllis gets along with her parents, and so on. What they will do, of course, depends to some degree on their economic prospects. It is undeniable that changes in AFDC over the 1960s made it marginally easier for Harolds and Phyllises who wanted to set up housekeeping while remaining unmarried to do so. The question is how the Harolds and Phyllises of the world responded to these marginal incentives, given that other arrangements would have made them better off economically and that other social and cultural variables bearing on their decisions were changing simultaneously. Murray's simplistic and distorted story gives us no answers to these questions.

Is there any way that we can determine whether the marginal change in the economic situation that Harold and Phyllis would face when receiving AFDC in 1970, as against its receipt in 1960, has had any substantial impact on the indicators of dependency that concern both Murray and us—illegitimacy and unemployment? Happily, the answer is yes. Although the state-federal arrangement for the distribution of Aid to Families with Dependent Children may have its drawbacks from the standpoint of national social welfare policy, it has great advantages for the measurement of the effects of different welfare policies on the poor. The economic incentives provided to go on AFDC are radically different from state to state.

In 1989, for example, a family of three would have gotten a maximum grant of $118 a month in Mississippi. That same family would have been entitled to a maximum of $663 per month in California.[17] If Murray is correct about incentive effects, we should expect to find that the illegitimacy rates in states with very high AFDC payments would be greater than the illegitimacy rates in states with lower payments. But careful research fails to reveal any significant effect of AFDC levels on illegitimacy.[18]

Perhaps Murray's thesis is not that absolute levels of AFDC benefits control illegitimacy rates, but that the rate of change in those benefits is determinative. If so, the data again fail to support his position. In the period 1960 to 1970, there is no consistent relationship between the rate of change in AFDC payments nationwide and the rate of change in illegitimacy.[19]

But Murray's thesis is not just about the level of benefits. It also concerns permissible living arrangements for welfare recipients. Assuming that the Harolds and Phyllises of the world

110

are prepared to risk prosecution for perjury and fraud, Murray expects that the elimination of man-in-the-house presumptions would discourage marriage and increase illegitimacy. There are two ways we might look for this effect. First we could look for an acceleration of the long-term trend toward higher rates of illegitimacy sometime in the mid- to late 1960s. But when we do, it is not there. The illegitimacy rate has been increasing since about 1950. There is no special kink in the curve in the late 1960s.[20] Another way to search for the Murray effect would be to look at the rate of illegitimacy for persons most likely to receive AFDC—teenagers, nonwhites, and high school drop-outs—against the rate for the population as a whole. Is there a blip in the late 1960s for those who would be most likely to respond to changes in economic incentives brought about by changes in AFDC? Again, no consistent effect can be found.[21]

In short, researchers have not been able to find any substantial evidence to support Murray's thesis that links increased illegitimacy to welfare changes. But what about unemployment or labor force participation? According to Murray's thesis, as the real value of AFDC benefits rises, more Harolds live off of more Phyllises' AFDC checks and become unemployed or drop out of the labor force. The reverse should also be the case—as AFDC benefits go down in real terms, the number of unemployed Harolds should decrease as well.

Testing this thesis is not as easy as one might think. The unemployment figures do not identify which of the unemployed are Harolds with a Phyllis to support them and which are the Homers who haven't a romantic prospect in sight. About the best that can be done is to look at the unemployment rates for young black men. Because black women receive about one-half of all AFDC payments, we are here in something like the right ballpark. But as the charts and tables in Murray's own book attest, the numbers moved in exactly the opposite direction from the one he would have predicted. As AFDC benefits went up in the late 1960s, the unemployment of young black men fell. As the real value of AFDC benefits declined over the whole of the 1970s, the unemployment rates for young black men rose.

The Simple but Bland Truth. Please do not misunderstand us. We are not asserting that there are no Murrayite Harolds and Phyllises out there. Like Murray, we believe that if you give people money, enough of it, they will, to some degree, reduce their work effort. We also believe that people who do not want to be married to each other, whether they have never been married or are married currently, will be somewhat more likely to remain separate or get a divorce if that choice does not make them destitute.

Our point is that Murray's story of the dynamics of welfare and dependency is wildly exaggerated. The change in economic incentives produced by the welfare "reforms" of the 1960s were quite modest, and the effects of those incentives on behavior were so small that serious social scientists have been unable to detect them after assiduous effort.

But if Murray is right that the latent poverty rate was going up during the 1970s and 1980s, and if we are right that this increase in "dependency" cannot be ascribed to American welfare policy, then what was happening? The answer is quite straightforward. First, pretransfer poverty is highly sensitive to the unemployment rate. Take a look at figure 4.3. The poverty rate for most periods parallels the unemployment rate. Indeed, serious attempts to estimate the impact of unemployment on poverty rates find that an increase in the unemployment rate of 1 percent increases pretransfer poverty by 0.7 percent.[22]

Second, demographic trends also affect the poverty rate. Certain groups—the aged, children, female-headed households, and nonwhites—have always been at greater risk of poverty in the United States. If the percentage of residents having these characteristics was increasing over the period from the mid-1960s to the mid-1980s, one would expect the poverty rate

112

WELFARE, POVERTY, AND THE WELFARE STATE

Figure 4.3   Unemployment Rate and Pre-Transfer Poverty
Rates, 1967–1986

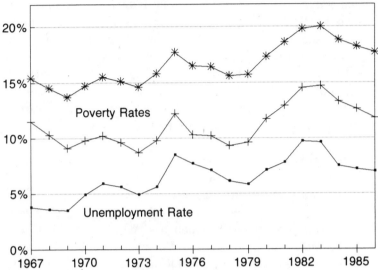

SOURCE: George Slotsve, "A Supplement to the Trend in Poverty,
1967–1985, Tables from the Current Population Survey," June 1986, revised
February 1987, revised May 1988 by Thomas Donley. Institute for Research
on Poverty, University of Wisconsin. Unemployment rate from *Handbook
on Labor Statistics*, August 1989, table 26, p. 129.
*Poverty rate, all nonelderly persons
+Poverty rate, all nonelderly persons with children under 18
• Unemployment rate

before transfers to be increasing as well. This has indeed been
the case. When the poverty rate for all persons is adjusted for
changes in demographics, it falls nearly 1½ percentage points
below the official poverty rate reported by the Census Bureau.[23]

Finally, a trend toward increasing inequality in earned income has been at work in the United States for the past several decades. Through the mid-1970s this trend was counterbalanced by the equalizing effect of rapidly rising income transfer benefits. But as the growth in social welfare spending slowed, the underlying tendency toward increasing inequality began to predominate. The causes of this trend are not well-understood, but it has been very broad-based, affecting virtually all population groups, occupations, and industries. It has not been limited to the poor but instead appears to reflect a trend towards inequality in the distribution of market income generally.[24]

These three factors—rising average unemployment rates, an increase in the percentage of the population in high-risk groups, and a long-term trend toward inequality in the distribution of market income—explain virtually all of the change in pretransfer poverty rates which has occurred in the United States from the beginning of the War on Poverty to the publication of *Losing Ground*. There is little cause for comfort in the identification of these trends. They pose a series of daunting challenges to policymakers. But we can at least feel confident that our efforts to relieve poverty have not been causing it to grow.

POVERTY, WELFARE, THE UNDERCLASS, AND WELFARE REFORM

Welfare is not causing poverty, illegitimacy, and a flight from work. But overall poverty rates are as high now as they were in the late 1960s; illegitimacy is increasing; and the employment rates of some subgroups, particularly of young black men, lags far behind the general population. The homeless on the heating grates and seeking shelter in the subways and other public spaces have brought the plight of the "down and out" forcefully to the attention of most Americans. In the press and elsewhere, we are told that a serious poverty problem exists and that its character has changed. It is increasingly difficult to view poverty as a temporary economic reversal in the life cycle of families. Instead, the emerging image of poverty is one of permanent deprivation combined with serious social pathology; it is a vision of what has come to be called "the underclass."

Who is this underclass about which there is so much concern? As definitions vary, so do the estimates of how large the underclass might be. At the most inclusive end of the spectrum of meanings are families who could be described as persistently poor. On that definition, we are talking about as many as eight million Americans. But, "the persistently poor" is a very inclusive description of the underclass. At the more exclusive end of the definitional range, the underclass has been described as including only individuals living in areas of extreme poverty (defined as a poverty rate of 40 percent or more) who are either working-age males not regularly attached to the labor force or household heads receiving public assistance. If that is one's vision of the underclass, then about half a million Americans fall into the category.[25]

Whatever the size of the underclass, it is the social problems besetting the neighborhoods in which they live that excites public concern—low rates of educational attainment and traditional family formation combined with exceptionally high rates of poverty, unemployment, illegitimacy, substance abuse, and crime. This is a vision of clusters of desperate people living in socially and physically destructive environments—people whose lives are substantially divorced from mainstream America. Their presence excites not only our desire to ameliorate suffering but also our fear of the dispossessed. Moreover, families facing all of these difficulties present a daunting challenge to policy reformers. What sorts of social policies would have any chance of making real progress against this synergistic melange of disadvantages?

This is not the place even to attempt to specify a grand strategy for coping with the underclass. The one thing that is clear, however, is that the major programs of the American welfare state have little impact on this group. Female-headed families with illegitimate children may, of course, be assisted by AFDC and perhaps by Medicaid, Food Stamps, and housing assistance. There is, in addition, a small special nutrition program for pregnant women and small children. However, unattached individuals and couples without children are likely to be ineligible for any cash benefits. Welfare state attention to their plight is demonstrated largely by their eligibility for Food Stamps, although SSI and Medicaid are available to some. Beyond that, the remnants of our always-modest-and-now-quite-small training and placement programs might provide some help. Substance abuse programs and the criminal justice system attempt to minister to the needs of others. This is clearly not a group of Americans for whom the welfare state has attempted to do a great deal. We may be blameworthy for our failure to attend more to the needs of the most disadvantaged among us. But this is evidence of a *gap* in our welfare state, not of the *failure* of welfare state programs.

Yet we can hardly resist making some collective effort to fill this gap, particularly where the victims of our inattention include large numbers of children. To do nothing to make their lives better, to provide no exit from intergenerational cycles of poverty, is to deny one of the fundamental principles of our insurance-opportunity state. Indeed, it may be that we should think of birth in disadvantaged circumstances as one of the risks against which the welfare state should provide insurance.

Something like this insurance view of the protection of children in poverty seems to be the animating vision of an essay by Daniel Patrick Moynihan published in the *New York Times* on September 25, 1988. That article was a public exhortation to Moynihan's colleagues in the Congress to pass his welfare reform bill, the conference version of the Family Support Act of 1988, which was about to be laid before them.

Moynihan begins by making several connected points about the current condition of children.

To talk about the condition of children is, by definition, to talk about the families in which they live. That is why we are going to have to learn to talk about two kinds of children, because—of a sudden, in a flash—we have become a society divided into two kinds of families. Call it a dual family system. In this dual family system, roughly half our children, somewhat randomly, but inexorably, are born without a fair chance.[26]

Moynihan goes on to describe the dramatic shift in the structure of the American family and the impact of this shift on children. Over half of all American children will spend part of their childhood in a single-parent family. And these single-parent families experience a very high incidence of poverty. Currently one child in four is born poor and, over time, more than one in three will, at some point, be on welfare. Because the economic fate of these children depends on family circumstances beyond their control, Moynihan characterizes child poverty as simply "a form of bad luck."

Moynihan notes that this bad luck has a tendency to repeat itself across generations. He cites evidence that daughters of single parents are 53 percent more likely to marry as teenagers than daughters raised in two-parent families. They are over 100 percent more likely to have children as teenagers and 164 percent more likely to have a child out of wedlock. Those who marry are nearly 100 percent more likely to divorce than are the daughters of two-parent families. The deprivations suffered by children in impoverished single-parent families make it much more likely that they will become the parents of such children in the next generation.

Moynihan argues that recent changes in our taxing and spending patterns, which have shifted income from the poor to the rich, work against providing a fair chance in life to every

American child. But he explains that the "greatest obstacle" to a fair chance is the current welfare system—by which he means Aid to Families with Dependent Children. Excoriating AFDC as an anachronistic program, originally designed for widows and orphans but now supporting a "wholly different population," Moynihan concludes:

In the next two weeks in Congress, we could secure the first real change in welfare since the program began. Both houses have enacted measures that respond to the new dual family system. We would take the present maintenance system and turn it into an employment program, with child support from absent fathers, transitional child care and health benefits for leaving welfare and unprecedented automatic funding for education and training.

A mother cannot work without child care. A mother cannot work without skills. The cost of providing these is manageable: 3 billion dollars to 4 billion dollars. The cost of not doing it is far greater and unacceptable: Every other American child will be born into a single-parent family, born to bad luck; every third American child will be doomed to spend part of his childhood on welfare, in poverty. In less than twenty years, these children will have children of their own. And so forth.[27]

Moynihan's "dual family system" is an even broader version of the underclass idea. Certain social characteristics determine not only a family's current economic success but also the probabilities of future success of its members. According to Moynihan's exhortation, the Congress should come to the rescue of these families and children. Welfare reform, the first real reform since 1935, will break this cycle of poverty and give American children a fighting chance for economic success. Reform will take the "employable" and make them the "employed." Work is to be required and assistance given in ways that encourage and promote work effort. In addition, absent fathers are to be made to pay support for their offspring.

Moynihan's rhetoric is characteristic of what has been said

about the Family Support Act of 1988, not only by its partisans, but by the press as well. This is presumably a bill that gets tough with both welfare mothers and absent fathers. But, as New York's former mayor, Ed Koch, liked to describe his own political stance, it is "tough love." Only by forcing the employable mothers of children on welfare to go to work and the irresponsible fathers who abandon them to pay for their support can we break the intergenerational cycle of poverty that consigns these children, and probably their children, to lives of poverty and desperation.

We believe, with Moynihan, that the Family Support Act of 1988 moves in the right direction. It recognizes changes in the characteristics and needs of the AFDC population and tries to respond to those changes. It is likely that the act will help reduce poverty in the United States, at least marginally. But we do not believe that much of that reduction will come from putting welfare recipients to work. Nor do we think this bill will stem the rising tide of single-parent families or make the luck of being born into one much less bad. Moreover, it is extremely important not to confuse the underclass problem that Senator Moynihan describes with other formulations of the problem. Children in single-parent families constitute a much broader category than either the persistently poor or the persistently poor beset by a host of other social problems. And, although most AFDC families are one-parent families, most of them are not "underclass" according to the narrower definitions described earlier. In short, the Family Support Act will probably reduce poverty somewhat, and it may give Americans a welfare system that reflects their values somewhat better than does the current one. But it is unlikely to ameliorate the condition of the core underclass or to cause illegitimacy, single-parent families, welfare, or Charles Murray's "latent poor" to disappear. Let us elaborate.

First, the good news on the poverty front. The Family Support Act clearly will eliminate some poverty among two-parent families and the working poor. The act requires that all states broaden their AFDC eligibility criteria to provide at least six months of coverage each year to two-parent families where one member is unemployed (AFDC-UP). Because fewer than one-half the states now have such programs, this will unambiguously increase the incomes of a nontrivial, but still small, number of poor families. Moreover, the working poor who claim the Earned Income Tax Credit on their tax returns and obtain a "refund" larger than their tax liability will henceforth not have that amount subtracted from their AFDC benefits. Finally, child care and other work expenses of working AFDC recipients are to be covered in more generous forms than in the recent past. The Family Support Act of 1988 increases cash benefits to a small portion of the AFDC population. This, in turn, will marginally reduce the incidence of posttransfer poverty.

Second, the symbolism of AFDC's new form is more consistent with American beliefs about family and work than our prior welfare arrangements. After its 1988 amendments, the AFDC program can no longer be castigated as a program designed to reward illegitimacy, irresponsibility, and sloth. Nationwide, whole families in poverty because of long-term unemployment, not just single parents, will now be covered at least part of the time. In addition, states will be required to make very substantial efforts to collect support from absent parents and to regularize the award of adequate child support by their courts. The first line of support for children is to be family obligation, not state benefits. And just as mainstream norms now expect most mothers to work outside the home even when their children are in their preschool years, so it will be for AFDC mothers.

These aspects of the reform effort are important. Indeed, the Family Support Act as a whole should be viewed as a success on these poverty reduction and value conformity grounds. Yet, the act risks being regarded as yet another welfare failure because it is being associated in people's minds with the elimination of poverty, the underclass, teenage pregnancy, illegitimacy, unemployment, and the need for welfare payments themselves. These are probably not achievable goals through any set of welfare state interventions. They are certainly not achievable through the Family Support Act of 1988. Consider the reasons why.

Unemployment and Poverty. The principal determinant of poverty is unemployment, and of long-term poverty, long-term unemployment. This is true not only in the United States; it is what our Western European allies have found as well. Most of the developed Western nations have seen their levels of poverty creep up over the last decade along with their levels of unemployment. In the United Kingdom, France, Germany, and elsewhere, there is increasing talk of a permanent class of persons left out of the labor market. Many factors contribute to this emerging problem, but in every case analysts have found high unemployment rates to be the principal cause.

The requirement that welfare recipients participate in training programs (to develop their job readiness) and accept employment where available only partially addresses the unemployment problem of the United States and its allies. It addresses the supply side of the problem but not the demand side. Unless there is a demand for these workers—a demand expressed in wages sufficient to lift them out of poverty—education, training, and placement programs will not have any substantial effect. And there is very little if any evidence from our prior efforts at job training and placement that operating on the supply side has significant effects unless combined with policies that heat up the labor market. This is a market in which supply does not create its own demand.

To be sure, there are mismatches between supply and demand in labor markets that can be alleviated by training and placement efforts. But advertised openings for marketing man-

121

agers and computer programmers are not going to be answered by welfare recipients who have just passed their high school equivalency exam. Nor are educationally less-demanding jobs available in the suburbs going to do the inner-city and rural poor much good. Improved training and job matching will help some but will not put most welfare recipients to work.

Moreover, the commitment to mandatory training and placement in the Family Support Act is quite modest. States will be required to provide work activity for only 40 percent of two-parent families in 1994, rising to 75 percent in 1998. But such requirements are expected to affect only about 6 percent of the total AFDC caseload.[28] The goals for single-parent families, who constitute the other 94 percent of the expected AFDC caseload, are far more modest. States will be required to provide training and placement assistance to a mere 7 percent of their nonexempt caseload in 1990, rising to only 20 percent in 1995.[29]

It is possible, of course, that states will eventually provide training and find jobs for all able-bodied AFDC parents by concentrating their attention on 20 percent of their caseload at a time. But this rosy picture is surely an illusion. After all, we have been here before. The rhetoric of its partisans aside, the newly named JOBS (Job Opportunities and Basic Skills) program that the Congress enacted is but an amendment to the existing WIN (Work Incentives) program that has been in existence since 1967. Many, many recipients have been enrolled in WIN, but the majority of them spend most of their time in a category called "holding." That is, they wait for appropriate slots to open up in one or another education, training, or placement program that might provide services to them. To be sure, the Family Support Act authorizes funding for the JOBS program at higher levels than WIN. But when lack of space is combined with the many legitimate exemptions from the program, it seems unlikely that the JOBS program will make massive strides beyond its predecessor in moving AFDC recipients into productive employment.

Again, do not misunderstand us. We are not arguing that Congress should not try to train welfare recipients for productive employment. Our point is merely that the program actually enacted is too modest to have a major impact. Its likely success in dealing with long-term poverty and unemployment for the AFDC population has been wildly oversold by its advocates. We must recognize further that it is a spectacularly underinclusive program in relation to the long-term poverty population. Only about half of the single-parent families in poverty receive AFDC. And the huge problem of unemployment among young black males remains largely untouched by AFDC and its new emphasis on work effort.

Illegitimacy and Poverty. To the extent that child poverty is the product of illegitimacy and the single-parent family, it is far beyond the power of the Family Support Act to control. One could describe the statute as telling Harold he will not get away with abandoning his illegitimate kids and Phyllis that she cannot expect to be a single parent "at leisure." Indeed, symbolically it does so. But it would be wrong to expect the Family Support Act to reshape the trend away from marriage and toward illegitimacy and single-parenting. These trends have been evident in the United States and in most European countries across all population groups and income levels since the early 1950s.[30]

Indeed, because these trends have been developing for several decades in countries having very different policies for the redistribution of income, it seems highly unlikely that marginal changes in one of our income transfer programs will have any significant impact. The population at risk is likely to continue to grow for the foreseeable future. It is almost impossible to identify or predict, much less to control, the cultural shifts or other changes that might alter this forecast. Meanwhile, we can make both welfare benefits and eligibility conditions more generous, reducing somewhat the posttransfer poverty of single-parent families. With a tight labor market, generous child allowances, health care, day care, and job training, we, like the Swedes, might control the incidence of child poverty and put virtually all parents to work. But the notion that the welfare reforms of 1988 are going to force Harold and Phyllis to the altar or make most families headed by Phyllises both fully self-supporting and free of poverty is a flight of fancy.

THE STATE OF WELFARE

"Welfare" (meaning the major means-tested programs of the American welfare state) has changed rapidly in the United States over the past two decades. In the late 1960s and early 1970s, welfare grew, both programmatically, adding Medicaid, Food Stamps, and SSI to long-standing public assistance programs, and fiscally, as Congress and state legislatures beefed up their attack on poverty. Since the mid-1970s, "welfare" funding has varied from program to program and within discrete periods, but the overall total has remained roughly constant. Meanwhile, economic conditions have worsened and eligibility requirements have become increasingly stringent. Welfare expenditures are a modest part of the welfare state, but the one most sensitive to the general economic health of the country. This sensitivity constrains the antipoverty effectiveness of means-tested programs. As poverty increases in bad times, welfare expenditures are unlikely to fill the gap.

But welfare cannot in any event be expected to eliminate poverty in the United States. Our welfare programs are not designed for that purpose. They are designed instead to support particular populations subject to risks beyond their control, and to provide certain basic goods and services necessary to health and potential productivity. We seek to protect the "deserving poor" and to provide the means for achieving economic self-sufficiency. It is both unnecessary and inaccurate to explain the failure of welfare to eliminate poverty by asserting that welfare *causes* poverty. The purpose, structure, and fiscal dynamics of welfare are explanation enough.

To evaluate welfare by its capacity to solve the pretransfer poverty problem borders on the absurd. Welfare's success or failure can be appreciated only in terms of its real aims—to help those who cannot help themselves and to promote family independence and self-support. Where those two aims are not perceived to be in conflict, as with support of the aged and the disabled poor, we have made real progress in reducing the incidence of posttransfer poverty. This progress is due, in part, to the greater fiscal stability of the welfare programs that target these groups (SSI and Medicaid), but more importantly to our relatively generous and nearly universal social insurance programs. On the other hand, where a conflict is thought to exist between the goal of relieving material distress and that of encouraging self-sufficiency, as in AFDC, we are prone to failure. We want to protect dependent children, but we do not want to encourage their able-bodied parents to abandon their responsibility to support either their children or themselves. The result has been a program with low payments and stringent, often degrading, eligibility conditions, a program that seems to serve neither of the purposes of welfare very well.

It is against this backdrop that we believe Congress's most recent efforts should be judged and approved. The level of childhood poverty has become truly alarming. The only reasonably sure way to protect dependent children from poverty is to see to it that their families receive more money. And the only way to provide more money without reducing parents' incentives to become self-supporting is to link increased payments to increased support for work effort and self-improvement.

Our expectation, as noted earlier, is that the "new" emphasis on work will not have big payoffs for the most disadvantaged portion of the AFDC population. But that is not an argument against trying, particularly where trying is the political precondition for making some progress on childhood poverty. Our fear is that this reform, like all of its predecessors, will ultimately be judged a failure because it did not accomplish goals that were beyond its reach (the elimination of poverty and welfare dependency) or because it did not resolve, once and for all, the conflict between insuring children against the risk of poverty while pressing their parents to become self-sufficient. This kind of evaluation is bound to undermine whatever good there is in the new conception of welfare's problems and options.

THE EMERGING AGENDA

The shifts in emphasis in the Family Support Act of 1988 will not, of themselves, solve America's problem with welfare, but they highlight two important ideas that together are likely to shape the welfare policy agenda of the next decade. The first is a willingness to spend more rather than less on welfare for the nonaged. The second is a policy focus broad enough to address the multiple determinants of a family's economic condition. In both instances the underlying political ideal is the opportunity side of the insurance-opportunity state. What may be new is the seriousness with which that ideal is being taken.

To take opportunity seriously requires that the conception of welfare be given an expanded and far more complex meaning. The 1988 act moves in this direction by acknowledging that an open-door economy is not a sufficient social welfare policy. Programs are needed to (1) equip clients to walk through those doors; (2) motivate them to do so; and (3) make sure that opportunity really is waiting on the other side. Moreover, these goals must be accomplished while recognizing that welfare programs confront economic, social, and cultural circumstances that can thwart the efforts of even those families best-equipped to succeed. To make progress, a complicated balance must be struck and maintained between the relief of individual distress, the encouragement of self-help, and the removal of systemic barriers to self-sufficiency.

This more complex vision of welfare policy quickly expands beyond welfare itself to include issues of education, crime, housing, and community development. It can, therefore, lead to a more sensible vision of what *welfare* policy alone can achieve and of what effective *social* welfare policy might entail. This "new" vision also has the advantage of consistency with our "old" ideals.

5

The Attack on Social Security

From roughly 1973 until the mid-1980s, the American public was treated to a steady diet of public handwringing about Social Security pensions. The first course in the standard fare of alarmist discussion was based on reports of projected shortfalls in Social Security's "trust fund," the system's bank account. "Bankruptcy" was predicted, and a Social Security "crisis" was announced. The main course consisted of a flurry of reform proposals deemed "absolutely essential" to avert disaster—proposals to reduce benefits, raise taxes, shape up administration, or perhaps all of these at once. For dessert, high anxiety was combined with pessimism as commentators complained that none of these needed reforms was likely to be enacted because selfish and shortsighted special interest groups had a hammerlock on the legislative process. The public was left with a heavy and uncomfortable feeling in the pit of its stomach. Images of fiscal crisis, instability, unaffordability, waste, and political deadlock began to spoil the sense of security the system was intended to provide. Indeed, an air of gloom came to surround almost any mention of Social Security.

In the late 1980s, America's public pensions were again front-page news. But the reason was not the familiar specter of "bankruptcy." Now the alarm was being rung for the very opposite reason—Social Security's trust fund was growing like Topsy. Positive balances amounted to some $70 billion and were projected to reach almost $12 *trillion* by 2030.[1] These projections are summarized in table 5.1.

The bizarre feature of the public commentary about this dramatic reversal of Social Security's fiscal fortunes was that the system's ever-resourceful critics—in the Congress, on television, and, most of all, in newspapers and magazines—responded to the news with the same fearful language they had used earlier to express dread of bankruptcy. The nation could "have a catastrophe waiting," worried one congressman, literally a "cri-

Table 5.1 Social Security Trust Fund Reserves,
Calendar Years 1985–2045[a]
(Billions of Dollars)

Year	Total Income[b]	Total Outgo	Annual Surplus or Deficit	Cumulative Reserves
1985	$ 203.5	$ 190.6	$ 11.1	$ 42.2
1990	309.5	252.2	57.3	211.9
1995	447.9	338.3	109.6	645.5
2000	631.5	446.8	184.7	1,409.4
2005	886.3	595.1	291.2	2,632.5
2010	1,237.9	825.8	412.1	2,632.5
2015	1,686.3	1,203.7	482.6	6,763.0
2020	2,226.2	1,775.4	450.8	9,124.3
2025	2,857.0	2,549.4	307.6	10,996.2
2030	3,590.7	3,524.5	66.2	11,837.5
2035	4,452.6	4,703.2	−250.6	11,240.0
2040	5,470.6	6,121.7	−651.1	8,840.4
2045	6,674.3	7,966.8	−1,292.5	3,799.4

SOURCE: *1988 Annual Report of the Board of Trustees of the Federal Old-Age and Survivors Insurance and Disability Insurance Trust Funds,* p. 64, table 23, and p. 141, table G1, Alternative II-B.
[a] Old-Age, Survivors, and Disability Insurance Programs
[b] Includes interest

sis of trillions . . . in slow motion," according to the editors of the *New York Times*. [2]

This is a strange fate to befall the most popular and successful social welfare program that America has ever launched. The language of crisis, which burdens our public discourse in so many domains, is particularly inappropriate in describing Social Security's past, present, and forecasted circumstances. Treating slowly developing trends as a "crisis" debases our political vocabulary. It scares citizens with cataclysmic images when they should be informed about choices, choices for which there is ample time for deliberation. Rather than presenting us with a crisis, our growing Social Security surpluses present us with important opportunities, along with certain risks that will have to be managed. They are certainly not dangerous circumstances somehow beyond our political control.

There is almost a surreal quality in the crisis-ridden concern about Social Security's surpluses. The doomsayers' basic worry seems to be that the proper amount of federal pump priming or fiscal restraint necessary to keep the economy humming will not be forthcoming because of the Social Security surpluses. Some critics fear that the surpluses will be spent, thereby resulting in too much government spending. Others fear that they will be saved, thereby resulting in too little spending. No one is bothering to ask why Social Security is cast as the culprit in this debate over fiscal policy. Social Security taxes and benefit payments are part of our overall fiscal and economic policies. What we do in this area certainly has effects on our overall economic health. But that hardly puts the Social Security program in crisis or makes it the cause of any other economic crisis.

Something peculiar is afoot in a polity where pundits see dire trouble no matter what the facts are regarding Social Security's deficits or surpluses. What explains this distemperate discussion?

Our basic conclusion is easily stated. For a substantial array of commentators, Social Security has become a scapegoat for anxieties engendered by a distressingly volatile economic environment. This volatility has forced us to make periodic adjustments in Social Security, and the problems of adjustment, always denominated "crises," have come to be located in the program itself. Had the country not faced stagflation from 1973 to 1983, fewer adjustments would have been needed, and the crisis rhetoric of the program's ideological critics would have had little impact. There is nothing in Social Security's politics, policies, or internal management that justifies crisis talk about the program. Moreover, the talk of crisis was always vastly out of proportion to the program's actual condition. Experience has shown us that relatively modest benefit reductions and tax increases, exactly like those enacted by the Congress in 1983, have been more than sufficient to produce short-run fiscal balance and, indeed, growing surpluses over the next quarter-century. Similarly, were we not preoccupied with the deficit, foreign trade imbalances, productivity declines, demographic shifts, and a host of other fears about the future, the news that surpluses were growing, that the Social Security system was in robust fiscal health, would not have been greeted with alarm.

In some contexts, public handwringing, peppered with cries of impending disaster, serves a useful purpose. It may be a necessary prelude to effective action. That is in some sense the story of Social Security reform in 1983. But when both fiscal famine and fiscal surplus are causes of equal concern, something has gone awry. The Social Security program itself has become a too-convenient target for displaced economic and social anxieties, hardly a benign development. Not only does Social Security–bashing distract us from addressing other relevant concerns, but it also breeds support for those who have always opposed the program. If long continued, a sense of crisis in and around Social Security could undermine public confidence and political support. And that truly would be a disaster.

Our aim is to defuse this sense of crisis and persistent malaise. A review of the characteristic criticisms of Social Security's durability and popularity shows that most of the critics' claims are simply false. Social Security demands thoughtful attention and can surely be made both fairer and more effective. But the issues facing it over the foreseeable future require, not dramatic changes in the program, but modest managerial adjustment. Beyond that, it is important to understand that the drumbeat of Social Security criticism to which we have been subjected since the early 1970s reflects an ideological bias that must be identified and confronted if discussions of Social Security policies are ever to generate more light than heat.

GENERATING FEAR AND LOATHING

What Americans Think. The typical American approves of Social Security but fears for its future. To understand and properly assess these feelings it is necessary to appreciate the peculiar nature of the public's knowledge of the program. Unless already retired (or widowed or disabled), the average American has little contact with the Social Security Administration (SSA), knows little about its program details, and would be hard-pressed to give even the barest outline of its scope, fiscal condition, or legal rules.

One result of this is that Social Security has a restricted meaning in America, in most people's minds referring only to retirement pensions. In reality, the term encompasses several contributory social insurance programs—old age and survivors' insurance (OASI), disability insurance (DI), and Medicare (HI) (collectively OASDHI). The more restricted popular vision has important effects on public consciousness. In Europe or Canada, social policy touches the lives of practically every family every month through child allowances and universal health insurance. In the United States, most working families experience Social Security only when they notice FICA's earmarked

deduction from their paychecks. Only a small proportion anticipate using, or actually use, the Social Security program's life
insurance or disability coverage before retirement. Thus, although Social Security is the most popular social program in
America, it plays a very modest role in our daily appreciation
of what American government does, and has done, well. And
"well done" surely describes the performance of Social Security
generally. Fifty years ago most Americans knew pauperized old
people, "on the county," as the expression went. The Social
Security Act of 1935 and its amendments over the years have
eliminated the equation of old age with poverty in the United
States.

At some level we all know this. Most of us have relatives or
neighbors who receive Social Security benefits. We vaguely
anticipate our own eligibility in the future and imagine that we
entitle ourselves to a deserved pension by "contributing" our
payroll taxes now. The survivor, disability, and health benefits
flowing through Social Security are acknowledged only when
we plan our life insurance coverage and as we approach our
own retirement. The result is a widely dispersed but intellectually thin attachment to the single largest collection of programs
in the American public household. Given their modest level of
daily exposure and programmatic understanding, it is remarkable how favorably Americans are disposed toward the Social
Security Administration as an institution and toward retirement pensions in particular. A program for which the vast majority of the population pay substantial taxes in anticipation of
receiving benefits decades hence does not seem like a natural
candidate for popularity.

Yet there can be no doubt of widespread support for Social
Security. Recent scholarship has documented what every sensible politician knows: Americans say they would pay higher
taxes rather than have these programs cut. Indeed, a 1986 survey of American opinion dramatically demonstrates both the
breadth and intensity of public support. More than four-fifths of

those polled (81.4 percent) expressed satisfaction with Social Security taxes. Nearly 90 percent of those satisfied were opposed to any spending cuts and 71 percent were willing to pay higher taxes to substantiate their commitment. Moreover, the intensity of the program's supporters—measured by a willingness to pay higher taxes or to write letters and sign petitions expressive of their views—was greater than the intensity of its detractors. As the authors of this survey note, Americans are overwhelmingly supportive of Social Security across race, class, regional, age, and partisan divisions.[3] Indeed, by a margin of approximately nine to one in all age groups, Americans want the Social Security program to continue. (See table 5.2.)

At the same time the public is undeniably apprehensive about the program's future. A majority in every age group below retirement age views it as at least "somewhat likely" that Social Security pensions will no longer exist when they retire, and among younger age groups that apprehension is overwhelming. (See tables 5.3 and 5.4.)

Why are Americans so fearful about the future of Social Security pensions? Social Security has not failed to make a payment in more than a half-century of operation, a fifty-year period that has included both war and peace, prosperity and recession, high unemployment and substantial inflation. The short answer is

Table 5.2   Support for the Continuation of Social Security by Age Group

	All Americans	Age 25–34	Age 35–44	Age 45–61	62 and Older
Should Continue	88%	88%	87%	89%	91%
Better to Phase Out	9	11	12	10	4
Not Sure	3	1	1	1	5

SOURCE: Yankelovich, Skelly and White, Inc., "A Fifty-Year Report Card on the Social Security System: The Attitudes of the American Public" a national survey conducted for the American Association of Retired Persons (Aug. 1985).

Table 5.3 Expectation That Social Security Benefits Will *Not* Be Available Upon Retirement by Age Group

	Nonretired Respondents	25–34 Years	35–44 Years	45–61 Years
Very Likely	28%	35%	29%	21%
Somewhat Likely	38	40	39	35
Somewhat Unlikely	19	17	18	23
Very Unlikely	13	7	13	19
Not Sure	2	1	1	2

SOURCE: Yankelovich, Skelly and White, Inc., "A Fifty-Year Report Card on the Social Security System: The Attitudes of the American Public" a national survey conducted for the American Association of Retired Persons (Aug. 1985).

Table 5.4

Confidence in the Future of Social Security by Age Group

	All Americans	Age 25–34	Age 35–44	Age 45–61	62 and Older
Very Confident	12%	4%	7%	12%	28%
Somewhat Confident	34	29	29	39	37
Not Too Confident	35	41	41	35	25
Not at All Confident	17	26	23	14	6
Not Sure/No Answer	28	37	25	6	4

SOURCE: Yankelovich, Skelly and White, Inc., "A Fifty-Year Report Card on the Social Security System: The Attitudes of the American Public" a national survey conducted for the American Association of Retired Persons. (Aug. 1985).

that for a considerable time, Americans have been regularly urged to be afraid.

Beginning in the early 1970s, a chorus of critics linked our undeniable economic troubles to Social Security. They forecast bankruptcy when what the Social Security program faced was simply the inevitable strain of reduced revenues (from unemployment, stagnant wage rates, and lower rates of economic growth) and unexpectedly higher benefits (from inflation's effect on indexed benefits). To cope with this fiscal strain, Social Security required (and got in 1977 and 1983) modest tax increases and benefit reductions. But the critics adjusted their vocabulary of alarm as events unfolded, always seeing cause for panic. They tried assiduously to turn the sacred cow of Social Security into something closer to an endangered species. The unreality of it all—the sheer foolishness of treating problems of adjustment as ones of impending catastrophe—got lost in the story. The media disseminated the tales of difficulty, finding it much easier to report the alleged crisis than to explain to the public that only small program adjustments were needed to correct Social Security's problems.

What the Critics Say. Who are these doomsayers? What precisely have these "nabobs of negativism," to use one of Spiro Agnew's colorful additions to our political lexicon, been up to in transforming choices into cataclysms? They are not simply right-wing demagogues, carryovers from McCarthyism who view the socialism of Social Security with the same dread they attached to communism in the 1950s. Nor is there some conspiracy afoot here. The critics are merely a contingent of conservative academics and popularizers of economic commentary, usually advocates of market discipline and strict limits on the scope of government, who accept society's obligation to maintain a safety net for the "truly needy," but who strenuously object to the government's providing income maintenance benefits to the middle class. Their aim is to do good, to set the record straight, and there are many aspects of their message that we should ponder as well as criticize.

Their major complaints about Social Security can be grouped under two headings: the dread of future economic troubles and the social waste of current and anticipated Social Security payments. The two concerns are connected analytically by the notion that eliminating Social Security's waste will also prevent the harm that the program does to the economy. They are also

linked ideologically by an often subtle but nonetheless important preference for "private," "individualist," and "market"
approaches both to the definition of social problems and to the
provision of government solutions. These critics constitute a
core cadre of residualists who oppose government social welfare benefits for anyone save on grounds of demonstrable poverty. In assessing their views of Social Security pensions, we will
first explore the analytic terrain and then attempt to map the
ideological roots of the multiple errors that have come to define
this intellectual landscape. A final section addresses what we
take to be a more reasonable set of concerns and opportunities
for reform.

Future Dread.   From a common starting point of concern
about the present state of the economy, almost all the Social
Security critics focus on the federal budget deficit and the vise
it has placed on the American public household. Agreeing that
anxiety about the level of the American budget deficit is warranted—and that tax increases are out of the question—they
look to reduced Social Security expenditures as the only remaining means of lowering the deficit. There simply isn't
enough "fat" to be found in other programs to get the deficit
"in shape."
   The connection between budget deficits and Social Security,
according to the most fervent advocates of fiscal prudence, is
simple and depends on facts with which we all can agree. The
federal government's outlays fall largely into four categories:
national defense, interest on the national debt, Social Security,
and federal medical care programs (Medicare, Medicaid, veterans' care, and so on). All the rest of the federal budget amounts
to less than a fifth of total spending. The smaller programs that
comprise the supposedly controllable portion of the federal
budget have already been cut substantially (in the 1981–86
period) and are too small, in any event, to constitute a major
source of deficit reduction. That leaves the nation very limited

choices: to reduce massive, well-defended programs or to increase taxes. Since tax increases are a last resort for most Republicans and Democrats, major program cuts are deemed essential.

No simple deficit reductions are possible in the portion of the budget devoted to interest payments. Interest due on the national debt must be paid. Since the amount due depends on the interest rate, which in turn partly depends on the size of the budget deficit, the only savings available in this area will flow from deficit reduction, not be its source. Prior to the precipitous decline of the Soviet military threat in the late 1980s, significant savings in the defense budget also seemed out of reach.

That leaves medical care programs and Social Security cash benefits as the only candidates for sizeable cuts. The one hundred billion plus federal budget for medical care undoubtedly contains waste, but no reasonable person believes that $20 to 30 billion of expenditures can be quickly cut from this area. Medical care cuts could help to reduce the budget deficit, but that still leaves the biggest program of them all, Social Security pensions. Those outlays represent some 20 percent of the federal budget and have been growing rapidly. Given these undeniable facts, the Social Security critics draw the seemingly plausible inference that, given the nation's trouble with deficits, the program must be reduced.

The conclusion that Social Security benefits must be reduced to cure our deficit ills took two forms in the late 1980s. Some commentators argued the case straightforwardly in the aftermath of the stock market crash of October 1987, urging congressional leaders to defy President Reagan's promise to keep Social Security "off the table" of budget negotiations.

Others expanded the deficit argument into a broader indictment of American economic performance, invoking the specter of economic doom to argue for a wide range of reforms, including a fundamental restructuring of Social Security. Peter Peterson's writings exemplify this genre. Peterson's basic arguments and alarmist tone are evident in his widely read 1987 article in *The Atlantic Monthly,* aptly entitled "The Morning After."[4] The country, we are told, "has let its infrastructure crumble, its foreign markets decline, its productivity dwindle, its savings evaporate, and its budget and borrowing burgeon." In consequence, a "day of reckoning is at hand."[5]

Social Security is implicated as the primary cause of our distress, but the attack is indirect. Peterson argues that Reagan's fiscal policy brought home the "hard" truth of the "law of unintended results." "In 1980 American voters decisively endorsed a smaller, leaner federal government, with special exceptions for defense spending and for poverty related 'safety-net' benefits." But we ended up "with a significantly higher level of federal spending in 1986 than we had in 1979" because of the inexorable growth of "entitlement programs".

Peterson's use of the entitlement category in this formulation and in the subtitle of his later book with Neil Howe is particularly interesting.[6] Social Security is politically popular. It is easier to condemn entitlement programs. This catch-all budgetary term lumps together the nation's social insurance programs (Social Security, Medicare, etc.) and its means-tested "welfare" programs (Medicaid, AFDC, Food Stamps, etc.). Since Social Security and Medicare make up the bulk of this category, the criticism is largely directed at them, but the critics' target is both masked and sullied by its association with the less popular means-tested programs. Thus, the familiar theme of social insurance's wastefulness is sounded without directly indicting Social Security.

At the same time, Peterson suggests there is something shameful and unsavory about social insurance benefits. They are characterized as "bluntly, welfare for the middle-class and up," which is "doled out regardless of financial need" (as if nonpoor persons did not have legitimate needs for retirement pensions, disability insurance, and medical care coverage in old age). The expression "doled out" has especially pejorative asso-

139

ciations. The "dole," a historical epithet for poor relief, has always been the most stigmatized form of public assistance. The term is surely inapplicable to contributory, non-means-tested, social insurance programs. Yet in one paragraph Peterson managed to link it with both Social Security and the nation's economic problems without quite saying so directly.

If deficits risk national disaster, any and all programs (as well as possible tax increases) should be on the table for discussion. In Peterson's words, we simply must "tame the federal budget deficit" to "reconstruct our future." We have been on a consumption binge, and we must pay off "our credit card bills." Where have we binged the most? You guessed it, the euphemistic "non-means-tested federal entitlement benefits," Peterson's evasive reference to Social Security pensions and Medicare.[7] Since the link between a consumption binge and the budget deficit is straightforward, it is a simple step to blame Social Security for a large part of the budget deficit and, with it, our other economic woes.

But has Social Security (as in the sense of old-age and survivors' pensions) contributed to the growth in the budget deficit since the reforms of 1983? The short and correct answer is that it has not; indeed the surplus of revenues over benefits and administrative expense has *reduced* the deficit from what it otherwise would have been. Look again at table 5.1. The Social Security surplus in 1990 will reduce the overall federal budget deficit by almost $60 billion. Over the next decade, the Social Security surplus is expected to grow to more than $180 billion a year. These surpluses are attributable largely to the Social Security tax increases enacted in 1983. Their growth is designed to pay the retirement costs of the baby boom generation that will leave the work force in the twenty-first century. It is these obvious facts that led Brookings economists Henry Aaron and Robert Reischauer to characterize Social Security as an "island of budgetary surplus in the midst of an ocean of red ink." On those grounds, write Aaron and Reischauer, "to suggest that

Social Security is part of the current deficit problem is lunacy."[8]

Could it be that the gurus of crisis do not know the fiscal facts? The answer is surely no. What they are arguing is that the economy is in such grave trouble that extreme measures are called for. They are not really saying that Social Security has caused deficit increases (they know better) but that there is no solution to the deficit problem without reducing Social Security benefits further.

The obvious question is why they do not recognize that Social Security surpluses have *already* reduced present deficit levels and will be reducing them more in the future. After all, assuming no other changes, the deficit would be even larger today without Social Security's contribution to national solvency. If Social Security is in fact the only fiscally sound portion of current federal budgets, exactly how is its spending taking us to economic hell in a handbasket? What exactly is all the shouting about?

The critics clearly have something more in mind than simple budgetary accounting. At this point the argument for a retrenchment in Social Security entitlements fragments into a series of concerns that are complicated, shifting, and interconnected. We will order the chaos by concentrating on three generic claims: (1) that Social Security decreases savings and overall economic growth; (2) that Social Security masks the true budget deficit, thereby prolonging profligate public policies elsewhere; and (3) that Social Security has made promises for the future that are unaffordable, thereby burdening the next generation with a massive debt and destroying their chance for a prosperous life.

1. *Crimes Against National Savings.*   Concerns about American levels of productivity, private investment, and both private and public saving have become familiar elements of our economic discourse. Many worried that levels of net private investment, 6.9 percent of GNP from 1970 to 1979, were too low. The

141

critics, again taking Peterson as representative, are even more distressed "that we have ended up with by far the weakest net investment effort in our postwar history" (averaging 4.7 percent of GNP from 1980 to 1986). Productivity growth, a "feeble 0.6 percent yearly in the 1970s," fell to a "still feebler" level of 0.4 percent yearly from 1979 to 1986. Public savings have, of course, been negative: The federal deficit level in 1986 was 4.9 percent of GNP, absorbing some 90 percent of all private-sector net savings that year, and our "publicly held federal debt is nearly three times larger than it was in 1980."[9]

The impact of Social Security financing on savings has been the subject of intense and continuing dispute among the nation's economists. Most of the disagreement has been technical, lodged in arcane journals read only by specialists. Those who claim that Social Security diminishes aggregate national saving—represented preeminently by former Council of Economic Advisor's chairman Martin Feldstein—make a straightforward case.[10] Workers, they contend, regard their payroll tax contributions to Social Security as saving. The anticipation of Social Security pensions, reasonably enough, may reduce the extent to which such workers believe they must save on their own for retirement. On the other hand, the federal government, under our pay-as-you-go method of financing old-age and survivors' pensions, regards revenues from Social Security contributions like other tax receipts and spends them. Consequently, Social Security contributions are not channeled, directly or indirectly, through the nation's capital markets into productive investment that could finance future pensions. At worst, according to this interpretation, the nation's capital stock is "trillions of dollars smaller" than it would have been if our pension system were "fully funded," that is, based on actual savings reserved for the use of individual workers when they retire.[11]

This "worst case" interpretation is wildly exaggerated. There is, in fact, scholarly evidence supporting all three possible effects of Social Security financing on national savings rates—that is, that Social Security affects the savings rate positively, that it affects it negatively, and that it has no net effect. In truth, the effect of Social Security on private savings is mixed. It is certainly the case, as thoughtful critics of Feldstein concede, that "OASI taxes displace some voluntary savings."[12] A number of private pension plans, for instance, explicitly reduce their own contributions in response to Social Security benefit increases. On the other hand, the knowledge that Social Security provides a reasonable floor under all retirement incomes may encourage savings as well. Because of the independence and security that Social Security promises to ordinary low- and middle-income workers, the nonwealthy may view retirement with greater optimism. If this is so, it makes additional savings to provide comfort, diversity, even luxury, in old age more attractive. Social Security may also encourage additional saving by the elderly themselves. Substantial numbers of middle- and upper-income retirees do not "consume all their [private] pensions during retirement," but instead save against the risk of catastrophic medical bills and nursing home stays, "knowing," as Nobel Laureate James Tobin rightly notes, that "any unneeded amounts will end up in their estates."[13]

Finally, it is far from certain that workers would actually save what they now pay in Social Security taxes if the present system were abolished. Many workers are so constrained by their present financial circumstances that they would be unable to save more even without the FICA tax bite; they would simply spend the added dollars on more pressing and immediate needs. Social Security's "forced savings" may be greater than voluntary savings would be in the program's absence. In fact, nobody really knows what Social Security's net effect is on national private savings. If that effect is negative, it is, "at most much smaller" than Feldstein's frightening estimates.[14] All that can be asserted unequivocally is that the experts do not agree that Social Security substantially reduces national savings.

If the expert consensus is as we have suggested, Social Security remains innocent of the charge of high crimes against national savings. Nonetheless, one might ask, is it not obvious that cuts in Social Security—or increases in its taxes—would reduce the net federal deficit and diminish the government's need to contract additional debt, thereby freeing funds for private investment that the government would otherwise have to borrow. This view—known as the "crowding out" hypothesis—certainly has some truth to it. A lower deficit would reduce the demand for funds in the capital markets and help to lower interest rates. In short, more public saving in government accounts would reduce the cost of capital and promote private investment.

Notice, however, that Social Security's current and rising surpluses are just such a move—an increase in taxes that reduces current consumption and increases overall savings. Notice, further, that all the talk about Social Security's effect on savings has in fact been about "private" savings. We can also save in our public accounts. These "public savings" have exactly the same effect on investment and economic growth as savings in private accounts. The traditional investment of Social Security's surplus or reserves in Treasury bills is irrelevant to the effect of public savings on private investment. Whether public or private, the effect of savings on investment operates through its effect on the supply of lendable funds, and therefore on the cost of capital. Additional Social Security reserve dollars bidding for Treasury issues has precisely the same effect on interest rates as does the same number of additional private pension dollars looking for a home. A belief that savings in private pension plans contributes more to investment and productivity than forced savings in the Social Security retirement account is either seriously misinformed or finds its support in theology rather than economics. *The only clear, current effect of Social Security surpluses, therefore, is to increase the net national savings rate.*

2. *Surpluses as Camouflage.*   The undeniably positive effect of the Social Security surplus on national savings has been challenged by adding a political analysis to the purely economic analysis of the preceding section. Social Security is but one contributor to public savings or dissaving. If Congress uses the Social Security surplus to mask deficits elsewhere, then we may have less public saving than the public actually wants and also less than would be produced by some other form of savings less easily used to camouflage other budgetary deficits. Moreover, there is evidence suggesting that just such a political con game has been in progress. Both President Bush, in projecting a balanced budget by the end of his first term, and the Congress, in meeting its yearly Gramm-Rudman-Hollings deficit reduction goals, use the Social Security surpluses to offset continuing deficits elsewhere.

As figure 5.1 shows, if Social Security is not counted, the federal budget deficit is actually growing (in nominal terms). Only by including the Social Security surpluses in their accounting can the administration and Congress make it appear that they are gradually taming the deficit monster.

But this so-called budgetary shell game has an obvious remedy—take Social Security accounts out of the general budget for purposes of meeting Gramm-Rudman-Hollings targets, establishing separate budgetary targets for general funds and the Social Security trust funds. Then the public will be better able to appreciate how much budget-balancing is taking place and whether it wants more or less of it. Indeed, the current unified budgetary reporting system risks misleading us about a number of things at once. It suggests more general revenue belt tightening than is actually the case. It uses a popular program's (Social Security's) quite different tax structure to finance indirectly current expenditures for purposes that have nothing to do with pensions and should be financed from other sources. Finally, it suggests a capacity to avoid future tax increases and additional public borrowing, when we are eventually going to have to do

Figure 5.1 Projected Federal Budget Deficits, 1990 to 1995
(billions of dollars)

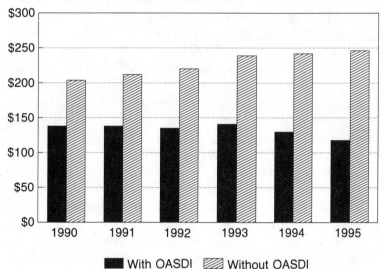

SOURCE: Congressional Budget Office, *The Economic and Budget Outlook: Fiscal Years 1991–1995*, January 1990, table II-6, p. 50.

one or the other to pay back what we are presently borrowing from the Social Security trust funds.

Notice again, however, that none of these concerns has anything to do with problems within the Social Security program. Each is a matter of budgetary reporting or political maneuvering in which the Social Security program's robust fiscal balance and current contributions to net national savings are being used for other, non–Social Security purposes. To view this situation as a problem *with* Social Security, or as a means by which the Social Security program promotes dissaving, is ludicrous.

Yet we are virtually certain that a way will be found to make the Social Security system the scapegoat. Indeed, that has already occurred. Responding to Senator Moynihan's proposal to reduce FICA tax rates in order to stop Congress from financing other expenditures with social insurance funds, *The Wall Street Journal* begins by attacking not the Bush administration's intransigent and profligate refusal to countenance any increase in taxes, but the myth of the Social Security trust fund. The *Journal*'s David Wessel says nothing that is false. But the tone, set by the opening sentence, is undeniably alarmist: "No, Virginia, there is no sacred Social Security trust fund in which your contributions are building steadily for your retirement."[15]

3. *Beggaring Future Generations.* Only the charge that Social Security pensions threaten to place unwarranted and unaffordable burdens on the next generation has sufficient substance to merit extended discussion. But, here again, it is not easy to keep sensible worries separated from runaway rhetoric. Moreover, the critical claims are quite varied, ranging from dire demographic projections to Peter Peterson and Neil Howe's claim that "the American concept of 'entitlement' [read 'Social Security'] is inherently prejudicial against the young."[16]

We shall begin with some straightforward projections. At present, for every person receiving Social Security benefits, there are three workers paying Social Security taxes. According to the "intermediate" projections of the Social Security's forecasters, the ratio of workers to pensioners will decline to about two to one by the year 2035. The ratio is projected to become even slightly more unfavorable before it improves sometime after midcentury. Assuming current FICA tax rates and making some further "intermediate" assumptions about economic growth and taxable wage rates, the trustees project very large surpluses building from now to about 2020 and then a spend down of those resources in the following three decades.[17] By 2050, the trust fund is projected to slip from surplus into deficit. These projections are illustrated in figures 5.2, 5.3, and 5.4.

Ignoring for now the question of how much faith to put in

Figure 5.2   Ratio of Beneficiaries to Covered Workers in
OASDI under Three Demographic Assumptions, 1970–2060
(Beneficiaries per 100 covered workers)

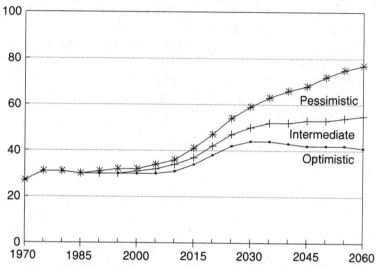

SOURCE: *1988 Annual Report of the Board of Trustees of the Old-Age and
Survivors Insurance and Disability Insurance Trust Funds* (Baltimore, Md.:
Social Security Administration, 1988), table 30, pp. 79–80.

seventy-five-year projections of either demographics or economic performance, this picture clearly permits critics to
choose their disaster—surplus or deficit—by choosing a time
period. Apart from providing grist for the crisis mongers' mill,
these projections suggest some issues for prudent political decision making. The obvious one is what to do about the post-2050
period when the Social Security surplus is projected to turn to
deficit. The less obvious one is how to pay back to the trust funds
the monies now being borrowed to finance deficits elsewhere
in the government's budget. According to the projections we

Figure 5.3 Social Security Trust Funds, Income and
Expenditures,[a] 1985–2045 (Percent of GNP)

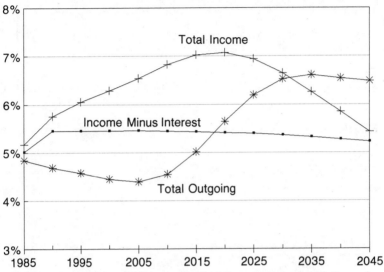

SOURCE: *1988 Annual Report, Board of Trustees, Federal Old-Age and
Survivors Insurance and Disability Insurance Trust Funds,* tables G1 and
G2, pp. 141–43.
[a]Total income consists of contributions, income from taxation of benefits,
interest income, and reimbursements from the general fund of the Treasury
for costs associated with special monthly payments to certain uninsured
persons who reached age 72 before 1968 and also have fewer than 3
quarters of coverage.
Total expenditures consist of benefit payments, administrative expenses,
net transfers from the OASI and DI Trust Funds to the Railroad Retirement
program, payments for vocational rehabilitation services for disabled
beneficiaries, and the special payments to the category of individuals
mentioned above.
The combined OASI and DI Trust Funds are estimated, under the
intermediate (II-b) assumption we are using, to be exhausted in 2048.

Figure 5.4   Social Security Trust Fund Reserves,[a] 1985 to 2045
(Percent of GNP)

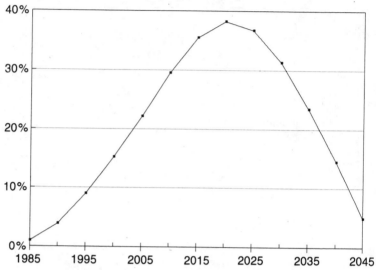

SOURCE: *1988 Annual Report of the Board of Trustees of the Old-Age and Survivors Insurance and Disability Insurance Trust Funds* (Baltimore, Md.: Social Security Administration, 1988), tables 22, G1, and G2, pp. 62, 141–43.
[a]Based on Alternative II-b

have reported, the Social Security system will have to begin calling in its loans beginning about 2020 in order to pay the pension benefits of the increasing number of baby boomers who will be retiring. How should we think about these issues?

Leading the attack, Peter Peterson and Neil Howe once again urge us to think about them in apocalyptic terms. They claim that "federal entitlement programs, as they are currently structured, will in future decades grow so large relative to our national economy that they will be patently unsustainable no matter how they are financed."[18] This is nonsense. To see why, we need only compare the share of net national product now devoted to all Social Security entitlement spending, including health care, with the share projected for the year 2060. As figure 5.5 shows, the amount goes from just under 6 percent in 1990 to slightly below 10 percent in 2060, a shift of 4 percentage points.

As we have said elsewhere, it is not clear what commentators mean when they say that programs are "unaffordable" or "unsustainable." But a shift of 4 percentage points spread over seventy-five years in the way net national product is expended can hardly qualify as either. This represents a projected annual increase of an infinitesimal four-hundredths of one percent. And, as Peterson and Howe themselves report, the percentage

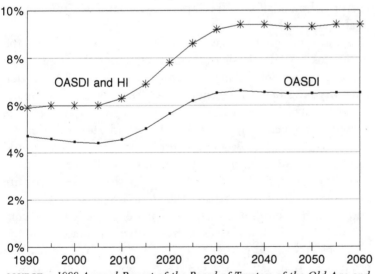

Figure 5.5   Social Security and Hospital Insurance Outlays 1990–2060 (Percent of GNP)

SOURCE: *1988 Annual Report of the Board of Trustees of the Old-Age and Survivors Insurance Trust Funds* (Baltimore, Md.: Social Security Administration, 1988), table F1, p. 136.

151

of GNP spent on OASDHI shifted much more dramatically than this in the period 1965 to 1986. Indeed, in that twenty-year period we went from spending 2.6 percent of GNP on these programs to 6.6 percent. Thus, in the last twenty years these entitlements have grown five times as fast as they are projected to grow in the future. The notion that the United States cannot over the next seventy-five years sustain a rate of growth in entitlement spending one-fifth that of the past two decades is preposterous.

Note also that the projected 4-percentage point shift in the utilization of net national product assumes, as do Peterson and Howe, that the programs and their expenditure growth rates remain unchanged. Looking again at figure 5.5, this presumption presents a very curious feature. It assumes that nothing will be done to tame the medical inflation that is fueling most of the growth: Two-thirds of the projected growth is in health insurance costs. In short, to the extent that Peterson and Howe are correct, the "unaffordability" problem is largely a problem of health costs—the subject of our next chapter.

If this is the situation as we can best anticipate it, how can the Petersons and Howes of the world unashamedly predict that Social Security entitlements will impose an impossible burden on the young of future generations? There are in fact many reasons, but chief among them is a general pessimism about the growth of the economy in the decades ahead. Henry Aaron and his colleagues at the Brookings Institution have demonstrated just how sensitive projected FICA taxes are to projections of economic growth. If real wages grow at the 1.4 percent rate used by the trust fund trustees in their projections, the total additional tax burden in 2060 is a modest 2 percent. If very pessimistic projections are used (based on our experience in the oil shock-stagflation period of 1973–85), the increased tax bite is a hefty 7 points, with the OASI share of combined employer and employee FICA taxes projected to eat up nearly 19 percent of payroll.

Because a 7-point increase in FICA taxes is less over seventy-five years than the 10-point increase experienced over Social Security's first fifty years, we have difficulty viewing even this pessimistic scenario with real alarm. We do view it with concern, however, because we fully agree with Peterson, Howe, and others that we are spending too few social welfare dollars on the young, and we fear, as they do, that a nearly 20 percent social insurance bite to fund old-age pensions might exacerbate this problem. Moreover, incremental increases in FICA taxes could stimulate nonincremental behavioral reactions affecting private savings rates, work effort, and so on. There may be some "perceptual thresholds" here that, once crossed, produce dramatic effects. On the other hand, as Lawrence Thompson said in 1990, "it is important to keep this . . . in perspective." Many European countries—notably West Germany—already bear pension burdens that approximate our forecasted strains without experiencing dramatically negative effects.[19]

The desire to stay in a tolerable tax range, however, does not require, or indeed justify, an attack on social insurance entitlements. It requires only a commitment to (1) prudent management of national economic policy to maintain growth and (2) a willingness to adjust benefit levels, the retirement age, and fiscal policies as experience teaches us what our real growth rates and our real willingness to pay increased taxes will be. Moreover, although prudence and a willingness to adjust expectations are often missing from our political practice and should never be taken for granted, they have not been alarmingly absent from Social Security policy-making. Indeed, the adjustments that have been made in Social Security since 1973 testify to the ultimate responsiveness of our political process when confronted with undeniable needs for incremental change. Further marginal adjustments in the retirement age or the portion of all wages subject to Social Security taxation could easily eliminate any significant shortfall in the trust funds that emerges over the next seventy-five years.

Prudent management of national economic policy is another matter. There is little disagreement among informed analysts that the fiscal policies of the Reagan years were profligate. The shift from "tax, tax, spend, spend" to "borrow, borrow, spend, spend" has produced a serious need for increased taxes that may or may not be forthcoming. But remember that in the land of deficit politics, Social Security is the only program in surplus. Moreover, if Congress either stops borrowing Social Security funds to cover its other current spending or spends more on human or physical capital that increases national productivity, then our Social Security surpluses will have been helpful. They will have contributed to a long-term economic growth spiral that reduces future fiscal burdens.

A 1989 General Accounting Office (GAO) report, recommending changes in our overall budget reporting practices, puts the matter well:

In this environment, current projections of future social security financing flows present both a challenge and an opportunity. The challenge is the burden of financing adequate benefits in a society with substantially higher ratios of retirees to workers. The opportunity is to use wisely the excess funds we now expect social security to accumulate over the next several decades. If they are used wisely, future incomes may be increased by enough that coming generations of workers will be able to support the higher number of aged citizens without suffering a decline in their living standards.[20]

The GAO report was, of course, much too moderate and sensible to be reported anywhere in the press.

Social Security's "Waste." The wastefulness argument is deceptively simple. Social Security wastes funds because it is "target inefficient," that is, because it makes payments to the nonpoor. Unhappily, this charge cannot be answered as succinctly as it can be made. Refutation requires an understanding that the critics' claim rests on both a misinterpretation of the fiscal facts regarding America's elderly and a misapprehension of the purposes of social insurance. Both the economic facts and the programmatic purposes are complex.

Critics of Social Security have made much of the improvement in the economic position of America's elderly since the early 1970s. "We can no longer afford to treat all the elderly as needy and special," writes *Newsweek*'s Robert Samuelson.[21] According to the *New York Times*, "one retiree in three [in 1959] lived in poverty; now [1987] it's one in eight, and the average retiree on Social Security has a higher average income than the rest of the population."[22] It is indeed true that the 20 percent across-the-board increases of 1972, coupled with the inflation indexation of Social Security benefits, sharply reduced measurable poverty among the elderly. The elderly's risk of poverty is now comparable to—indeed, slightly better than—that of other age groups rather than being much greater, as it was in earlier periods.

These developments have reduced poverty among the old; they have not created islands of luxury. Social Security's benefits are now decent, not grand. In December 1988 the average Social Security pension was $537 per month for retirees and $493 for aged widows and widowers. In real terms, these modest averages describe both the present and the foreseeable future. Moreover, Social Security is as crucial to the well-being of most of the retired as it is central to avoiding poverty among them. Social Security pensions make up more than half the income of 53 percent of the elderly. Many of the elderly are close to poverty under current circumstances; 8.1 percent of them have incomes less than 25 percent over the poverty line, compared with 4.7 percent of the nonelderly in that near-poor band of income. "Any large cuts in benefits," as Henry Aaron and Robert Reischauer rightly argue, "would push some of the [elderly] below the poverty threshold and return many to the position of economic inferiority from which they only recently emerged."[23]

As we noted in chapter 4, Social Security pensions are America's most effective poverty-reduction program. They keep more people out of poverty than any other government effort. They also support more of the near poor than any other program—indeed, more than all other programs combined. Why then is the program criticized for failing to target the poor rather than applauded for its successful prevention of poverty among the aged? The answer is that the critics of Social Security believe it could be a better antipoverty program if the reduction of poverty were its only purpose. Its failure to be only an antipoverty program necessarily means that it "wastes" billions on the nonpoor.

In one common form, this view expresses itself as a rhetorical question. In a world of strained public budgets and massive budget deficits, why should Social Security pay a dime to the Rockefellers? A *New Republic* article on "The Social Security Rip-Off" announced that it was "time we told the widow in the East Side luxury condominium that she's getting what amounts to welfare at the expense of the low-wage worker in the South Bronx."[24] Of course, there are not enough Rockefellers or rich widows to make a perceptible dent in Social Security's finances, but this obvious point is lost on the shrill critics of Social Security's waste. If the goal of humane social policy is to rescue the victims of capitalism, why waste resources on those who can easily help themselves? How can it make sense to do anything but target Social Security's massive outlays on the poor?

The charge of wastefulness in pensions (and social insurance generally) expresses more than a conviction that universalistic programs inefficiently meet the needs of the poor. The critics proceed from a fundamentally different notion of appropriate government purpose than that embodied in our social insurance programs. For these analysts—let us call them "poor-law residualists"—legitimate social programs exist solely to help those who would otherwise be demonstrably destitute. Residualists may well disagree about precisely which groups within the poor are deserving, but they presume that all social aid should be means-tested. Redistribution is legitimate, but only if its scope is strictly limited to those who can document a lack of adequate income and assets to support themselves. If one accepts this residualist view, then social insurance programs like Social Security are necessarily "wasteful."

But why should one evaluate social insurance retirement benefits by this targeting test? Few Americans accept the residualist standard for social insurance or want to participate in residualist programs (that is, receive "welfare"). In fact, the central rationale for social insurance is to *prevent* destitution, not to relieve it, to avoid the need for widespread residualist programs through the social insurance device of compulsory contributions and mass pensions. Indeed, according to the most optimistic aims of the 1930s, social insurance was to make sure that means-tested programs for the aged would wither away.

However phrased, these differences in evaluating Social Security are crucial to the claim of waste. To satisfy the principled residualist, public programs have to do the work of private charity more effectively and completely. For the principled advocate of social insurance, the test of success is whether the nation's citizenry is protected against sharp declines in living standards as a result of a breadwinner's retirement, unemployment, death, or disablement, and without having to submit to demeaning means tests or suffering a sense of estrangement from the mainstream of social life. No amount of data manipulation can resolve these differences. Lack of targeting—lamentable on residualist grounds—is praiseworthy evidence of success for social insurance enthusiasts. Put another way, target inefficiency (regarding poverty) is the very source of social insurance's widespread acceptance and political stability.

The debate clearly does not concern the facts of "waste" but rather the relevance of the social insurance and residualist standards in the first place. By assuming that universal programs are wasteful, the critics reveal their fundamental disagreement with social insurance's core assumptions. But it makes a big difference in political life whether a disagreement concerns the appropriateness of a particular goal or the appropriateness of a particular strategy for achieving an agreed goal. The critics of social insurance confuse the first kind of disagreement with the second.

The most persistent critics of Social Security waste have been fiscal conservatives who favor means-tested, residualist programs because they are small as well as "target efficient." However, neoliberal critics of government ineptitude have also adopted this line out of a genuine yearning for more generous treatment of America's poor. As the *New York Times* asked in a 1987 editorial, "why neglect a whole population's vital interests for the sake of affluent retirees?"[25]

This position is commonly linked to demands that social insurance be "means-tested." But by this something quite different is meant than the eligibility-restricting measures associated with AFDC. The neoliberal critics recognize that such practices would undermine Social Security's popularity by turning it into a "welfare" program. They define means testing differently, suggesting that we "treat Social Security payments as ordinary taxable income."[26] If Social Security—or the cash value of Medicare and disability insurance—were made wholly taxable, then higher-income Americans would receive lower after-tax benefits than is now the case. In the world of these neoliberals, the consequence would be greater progressivity in social insurance programs, an aim they share with many others across the political spectrum, ourselves included.

The difference between them and us lies both in substance and in tone. These critics often advance their position with a stridency typical of the recently converted. "The Elderly Aren't Needy" was the title of Robert Samuelson's controversial article on behalf of taxing Social Security benefits. His major assault on wastefulness consisted of the claim that "Social Security is a welfare program: Today's taxpayers pay today's beneficiaries. It's a great program that's created huge social benefits," Samuelson crows, "but it's still welfare."[27]

Convinced of the rightness of their sympathies and the foolishness of Social Security's most ardent Democratic supporters, the neoliberals sneer at the gap between their insights and those of Social Security's loyalists. "If the large and growing Social Security elephant remains free to graze where it pleases," the *New York Times*'s Peter Passell has written, "other public interests will be unjustly trampled."[28] Presumably both Samuelson and Passell are pursuing the same end—cutting Social Security down to size so that other social welfare goals can be accomplished. Samuelson whacks away with the "welfare" epithet, Passell with the image of a greedy elephant trampling over other, more worthy, social goals.

We believe such criticism to be both analytically and politically naïve. First, the analytic naïveté. That today's taxpayers pay today's beneficiaries is hardly enough to turn Social Security into welfare. To be sure, the term is a loose one having many connotations, but two things seem central to the American conception of welfare. The first is that poverty is a necessary condition for receiving payments. The second is that welfare benefits need not be justified by prior contributions to the program in question or to the economy generally. Neither of these features characterizes Social Security.

This analytic mistake leads to a political error that seems so obvious that we marvel at how common it has become. The assumption is made that once the public recognizes that Social Security is welfare or a greedy "elephant," it will decide to shift its financial support to the truly needy. This notion is decidedly peculiar. It seems to imagine that Social Security achieved its current size, structure, and popularity by accident or error. If people could be made to realize the true nature of the monster in their midst, they would see the good sense of doing things differently.

This is not a realistic view of the world. First, the public is highly unlikely to consider Social Security as welfare while paying FICA taxes and receiving universal non–means-tested benefits in return. "Welfare" simply does not describe the program that the public experiences. Second, should the public for some reason decide that Social Security *is* welfare, or is vastly and inappropriately overgrown, it need not, and almost certainly would not, decide to maintain the same level of benefits but redirect them to the truly poor. No targeted welfare program, including those for the aged, provides anything approaching Social Security's benefit levels. As the old saying goes, "Programs for the poor are poor programs."

Nor is there any reason to think that the public would be willing to pay the level of taxes it now pays through FICA to support some other set of "public interests" now being "trampled" by the Social Security elephant. If the public preferred some other set of interests to those served by Social Security spending, it is hard to see why so many politicians are so confident that the public does not want Social Security trimmed.

ERROR AND IDEOLOGY

Several conclusions seem warranted. First, there is no crisis in Social Security. The system is fiscally sound and immensely popular. Second, Social Security is not causing macroeconomic difficulties. Indeed, it is the only large government program currently making a demonstrable contribution to net national savings and thereby promoting investment through the reduction of the cost of capital. Third, Social Security makes the largest contribution of any major program to the reduction of poverty in the United States while avoiding the stigma and the political unpopularity of welfare. Far from being wasteful, this program is a major success.

We must therefore admit to a certain bewilderment as we compare the fiscal facts and the real public purposes of Social Security with the continuing chorus of commentary so critical of the program. The hostile criticism suggests a sustained failure of comprehension, not by a general populace understandably inattentive to these matters, but by otherwise well-informed commentators. To be sure, the nation's economic troubles have provided ample opportunity for government bashing, but why bash this particular program in these particular ways?

We think the answer is ideology. These critical commentators, despite their different claims and differing perspectives, share a private, individualist preference for market-directed activity. This position is understandably hostile to a social insurance conception that relies on government provision, features communitarian ideals of universalism and social solidarity, and uses the coercive legal instruments of taxation and entitlement to achieve collectively approved ends. Looked at through their ideological lenses, the Social Security program appears to be riddled with defects and inconsistencies, indeed, with myths and frauds foisted on an unwary populace. Analyzed from this perspective Social Security is a frightening political specter, and this fright seems to stimulate both hyperbolic characterization of potential future troubles and misconstruction of the program's current impact.

The ideological element in programmatic misanalysis is perhaps clearest with self-proclaimed libertarians like Peter Ferrara.[29] His complaints about Social Security fall under at least five headings: (1) its negative economic impact; (2) its unfair rate of return; (3) its coercive and uniform nature; (4) its regressive taxation; and (5) its lack of real security given concerns about its continuation into the distant future.

Ferrara believes that all of these difficulties result from the "inherent contradiction" of combining a welfare and an insurance program in one package. The inherent contradiction thesis need not detain us at this point. It rests on the essentially silly notion that programs have, or should have, only one purpose, and that any compromise among purposes within a program is evidence of a disabling "contradiction." We have already commented on the unhelpful character of this form of policy analysis in chapter 2.

The negative economic impacts that Ferrara asserts are of two sorts: one is the familiar "crime against national savings"; the other is the effect of Social Security taxes on work effort. Is there anything new in this? We have already explained why the crime against savings charge constitutes a bum rap. The only wrinkle to notice here is the inconsistency of this claim with Ferrara's fifth claim that the program provides no real security. If the latter were true, there should be no effect on private savings. If people believe they cannot rely on Social Security, why would they reduce their savings in response to it?

We have not previously addressed the other negative economic effect which Ferrara attributes to Social Security—a withholding of work effort in the face of Social Security taxes. It is hard to know what to make of this argument. If tax payments really do reduce work effort, there is no reason to single out Social Security taxes for special blame. One wonders what sort of tax system would not be subject to Ferrara's criticism. Apparently he favors a general lowering of taxes by the amount of the Social Security tax itself. If the tax disappeared, and with it, of course, the program, then people would receive more present income from their work and, according to Ferrara's logic, they would respond by choosing to work longer hours.

This effect of course depends on some crucial assumptions. At its core is the view that people do not believe they are getting their money's worth for their Social Security taxes and therefore regard those taxes as an uncompensated reduction in their real income. If people think they are getting good value in exchange for their payments, their work effort will not be reduced anymore than it is when they spend current income to buy a car. In short, Ferrara seems to assume that people see the system the same way he does—as providing an unfair rate of return through a coercive program that regressively taxes a current generation unlikely to receive benefits when its turn comes. This is, of course, inconsistent with the polling data that finds 82 percent of Americans highly satisfied with the Social Security program and 71 percent willing to pay more to maintain the program at its current level.

Ferrara apparently ascribes public satisfaction with Social Security to the quasi-fraudulent nature of the program itself—a "Ponzi scheme" that has hoodwinked the populace into believing in trust funds that do not exist and into accepting rates of return that border on theft. Even viewed from Ferrara's libertarian perspective, the "unfair rate of return" and "Ponzi scheme" characterizations are peculiarly simpleminded. The real annual rate of return on Social Security taxes for persons who will be taxpayers and beneficiaries over the next fifty years is estimated at about 2 percent. The historic return on Treasury bonds over the last fifty years has been somewhat less. A well-diversified portfolio of common stocks over the past fifty years has done better—approximately a 6 percent real return. However, there is a big dispersion around the average return on a stock portfolio in any given year—from minus 21 percent to plus 27 percent. The wealthy can afford to devote a portion of their assets to higher risk investments because they can afford to absorb the losses they may incur. A pension system designed to provide a secure income floor for a nonwealthy population cannot, or rather should not, incur a similar level of risk. Because the variability of return associated with the stock market is likely to be unacceptable in a basic retirement program, it is hard to see why the Social Security system's 2 percent real return should be characterized as "unfair."

A "Ponzi scheme" is a form of securities fund swindle in which the investments of new clients are used to pay dividends or redemptions to old clients—and, of course, a huge rake-off to the promoters—without ever investing the money in the securities markets. Applying the epithet to Social Security is to label the system's pay-as-you-go financing structure a fraud. It is, of course, no such thing. Nor would the promises of Ponzi scheme operators be fraudulent if, like the Social Security system, they had the duty and the means to make all promised benefit payments and had done so without fail for over fifty years. This characterization of Social Security financing amounts to nothing more than mud-slinging.

The coercion and uniformity about which Ferrara complains are the necessary features of a system that does not have a variable rate of return and also protects against free-rider problems. Arbitrary coercion should be avoided where possible, but here the use of state compulsion is amply justified. Foregoing current consumption to save for old age is often difficult. People engage in many strategies in an effort to force themselves to be more prudent in this regard. However, there is no contract one can make with oneself that is enforceable. The Social Security system merely enforces a form of self-paternalism that most people find useful, even if grudgingly so. The system's immense popularity attests to the public's desire to impose this discipline on itself.

There is, no doubt, a mild regressive taxation problem in the Social Security system. But that is hardly a reason to junk the entire scheme. Social Security taxes can and should be made less regressive. Moreover, the regressivity of Social Security taxes can be further moderated through adjustments in the general income tax system. A simple expansion of the earned income tax credit (EITC), for example, can provide a tax credit that effectively returns a portion of FICA taxes paid by persons having incomes below a certain amount, subject to a progressive phase-out as income increased. Indeed, this is precisely what was done in the 1986 Tax Reform Act.

Fear of the system's discontinuance is hard to allay. Fifty-year time horizons seem fanciful when applied to anything. The relevant question, however, is not "Do you feel secure?" but "Does this program seem as secure as other means of providing old-age pensions?" The answer to the second question is surely "Yes." Social Security's longevity, popularity, and malleability suggest that it is a survivor by comparison with any other program. The simple projection of demographic trends and unchanging rules into the distant future certainly suggests problems. But why should such a rigidly inflexible scenario be the basis for even a moment's discussion? In the 1950s and 1960s we had to find a way to house and educate the baby boom generation. In the 1970s and 1980s we had to integrate them into the labor force. In the next century we will have to support them in their old age. A population with a "lumpy" age distribution has to be flexible. Because the population's needs change over time, more schools are needed in one decade, more jobs in another, and more old-age pensions in another. None of these adjustments is easy, but nothing in the nation's history over the past four decades nor in the history of the Social Security program suggests that we are incapable of making the adjustments necessary to support the baby boom generation in its retirement.

Even in its own terms, Ferrara's argument is largely fatuous. But the important point for current purposes is the ideological consistency that structures his particular claims. Ferrara relentlessly characterizes the issue of retirement security as an issue of individual financial planning. He misanalyzes public fiscal arrangements (the pay-as-you-go Ponzi scheme) by giving them a characterization based on misleading private market analogies. He conceives of citizen choice as expressible only in uncoerced private transactions. He understands income redistribution only by analogy to private charity and social insurance only by analogy to private insurance. He thus cannot avoid concluding that the multiple purposes of Social Security are some sort of horrid mistake—or worse, a political shell game. Viewing social insurance through libertarian glasses is truly to see "through a glass darkly." An image of pervasive error is the predictable result.

Subtler but similar ideological commitments seem to undergird the misdirected worries of most of Social Security's other major critics. For example, Peterson and Howe's fixation on the dreadful consequences of promising entitlements without currently funded accounts to service the looming liabilities is understandable from a private insurance perspective. In the world of private insurance, contractual commitments (the entitlements) are indeed rigidly fixed for the future. The insurance company can make a credible commitment to pay its obligations only by amassing sufficient reserves to cover all contingencies. But this kind of rigidity describes neither the legal situation nor the statutory history of the Social Security program. Public entitlements can be modified, and the government has resources in its power to tax and to create money that lend credibility to its unfunded liabilities in a way that no private insurance company can match.

The seeming blindness of these authors to the equivalent effects of public and private savings on investment and to the spectacular antipoverty gains made possible by universal Social Security pensions may have a similar explanation. Peterson and Howe just cannot see Social Security surpluses as savings. Indeed, in their pursuit of increased private savings through reduced FICA taxes, they commit the same error for which they spend pages excoriating the Reagan administration—the belief that reduced taxes will translate into increased private savings rather than increased private consumption. In their patrician concern to construct a beneficent welfare system for the needy, they cannot see the stigmatizing effects that private charity and means-tested public assistance impose on recipients by so sharply distinguishing between the needy and the rest of us. It is precisely such distinctions that destroy the sense of shared rights and a shared fate which sustains the public commitment to social insurance and makes its antipoverty successes possible.

The misdirections of policy analysis that we have been examining are surely not accidental. Moreover, their ideological origins suggest a rather different dimension of trouble for the Social Security system. The critical commentators we have been discussing are not lunatics. Most are well within the mainstream of current political debates. Their ideological commitments are both coherent and familiar to many Americans, and their claims are not routinely challenged by analyses based on a similarly coherent and familiar ideology of state provision, social solidarity, and public finance. We run a small risk therefore of undoing a great American success story because we have forgotten what it was about.

WHITHER SOCIAL SECURITY:
AN INCREMENTALIST VIEW

For now we will rest content with the recognition that all successes are qualified. Social Security is hardly perfect. And more to the point, the economic uncertainty that has led to Social Security–bashing is not over. Economic troubles and demographic shifts may well demand additional adjustments in Social Security. We should, therefore, consider ways in which Social Security recipients can legitimately be called on to make a contribution to economic sacrifices that others in the society may be unable to avoid. Put another way, there are some sensible adjustments in Social Security that, in a less overheated debate, should be rationally considered. We will begin by discussing proposals that do not make sense and work our way toward some principles for reform.

Across-the-board reductions in benefits would be justified only if the Social Security program itself were excessively generous. And, although we can identify virtually no one who holds this view, there seems to be an attraction for one form of across-the-board cuts—reducing the annual cost-of-living adjustment (COLA)—which makes the least sense of any such proposal. The political attraction of COLA-tinkering lies largely in the partial invisibility of its effects. But consider the long-term consequences.

Some have suggested, for example, that Social Security benefits should be adjusted only when inflation exceeds 2 percent per year. The argument is that modest inflation hardly warrants concern and that large dollar savings can be found through this innocuous change, one that would affect all Social Security benefits. Small reductions in a large benefit total mean substantial budget savings—another way of saying that across-the-board cuts should be enacted.

But small changes over a long period add up to significant reductions that show up in peculiar places. The 2 percent formula, for example, would link benefit reductions, in effect, to age. The longer a recipient lived, the greater the benefit cut they would absorb. It would "ensure that the oldest and most vulnerable would suffer the greatest income loss." An 85-year-old widow would "receive benefits nearly one-third smaller than she received at age 65." A disabled 25-year-old's benefits would be cut in half by age 60. Such consequences justify the conclusion that "such a grotesque proposal deserves not serious debate, but derision."[30]

Proposals to limit cost-of-living adjustments to the *first* 2 percent of inflation would discriminate on the basis of age in the same way. In addition, protecting beneficiaries only from modest inflation would leave them vulnerable to the real calamity of rapid inflation. If the purpose of indexation is to maintain real levels of benefits in the face of inflation, tinkering with indexation adjustments should be approached with the utmost caution.

The indexation formula we now use, however, bears reexamination. Some argue, for example, that it wrongly adjusts for inflation in new housing when most of the elderly either already own their own homes or could not possibly do so. Others, like James Tobin, also argue that indexation should not protect any particular group from declines in national wealth.[31] The oil price increases of 1973–74 and 1979–80 provide good examples of Tobin's concern. The inflationary jolts caused by these price increases made the whole nation poorer. It is difficult to make a good case for absolving the elderly from sharing in this loss. Tobin argues for excluding certain inflationary elements from cost-of-living adjustments in Social Security as well as in other programs. In effect, this is a call for an improved price index. It suggests no rejection of indexation nor any erosion in our commitment to maintain the purchasing power of Social Security benefits. The issue raised involves the technically proper adjustment of accepted benefit levels, and that is an entirely appropriate and useful object of inquiry.

This is not to rule out changes in Social Security that could make a sensible contribution to reduced deficits (and greater social equity). We believe the most reasonable proposal along these lines is to subject a greater proportion of Social Security benefits to income taxation. At present, a portion of Social Security benefits is taxed if the recipient's income exceeds a certain threshold level. In 1989, 16.5 percent of all Social Security recipients were subject to this tax. Recipients with cash incomes less than $25,000 were not affected, and only about a third of recipients with cash incomes between $30,000 and $40,000 were affected. But almost all recipients with incomes greater than $40,000 were affected to some degree, and those with incomes greater than $100,000 effectively lost 15.5 percent of their benefits because of the tax. Altogether, 1.8 percent of all Social Security benefits were returned to the government through increased income taxes.[32] The Congress could increase tax revenues without unfairly burdening the least secure among the elderly by lowering or eliminating the income threshold above which Social Security benefits are taxed or by increasing the fraction of benefits subject to taxation.

Such policy changes have much to recommend them. If carefully crafted, they could make Social Security's tax treatment more comparable to that of private pensions; and they would permit the inclusion of Social Security in a broader deficit reduction compromise without reducing the incomes of the "large proportion of the retired population that is clinging precariously to its modest, but not sumptuous, standard of living."[33]

There is another reason, unrelated to budgetary concerns, why the taxation of Social Security benefits makes sense. Social insurance benefits—for retirement, for disability, for unemployment, or for the premature death of a breadwinner—are designed to replace the earnings on which families depended for their standard of living. They are substitutes for wage income, provided under circumstances that warrant general social protection. They function, in effect, as a means of continuing wage income in the face of contingencies faced by all families.

To the extent that social insurance benefits are regarded as wage replacements, it makes sense to subject them to income taxation. Viewed in this way, they look like part of the income flow that ordinary income taxation is meant to reach. Since the income tax system recognizes other sources of income besides wages and salaries and taxes income by a progressive formula, there is a strong case for including some or all of Social Security benefits in the definition of current taxable income. This approach is also consistent with basic principles of social insurance. We earn our place in the distribution of social insurance benefits by the consistency of our employment and the wage levels we achieve as workers. By this logic, it makes sense for benefits to be distributed as wage substitutes, subject to the same taxation as current wages.

Other considerations limit this argument's appeal. One is that most Americans perceive their contributions to the Social Security trust funds as coming out of already taxed income. The public simply does not view Social Security taxes in the way that it views federal income taxes, even though the only functional difference between them is that FICA tax revenue is reserved for designated purposes. It may be that the public wants FICA tax payments to feel like private pension contributions. If this is so, the tax status of those contributions is of more than purely fiscal concern. Viewed in this light, the fact that covered workers pay income taxes on their half of FICA contributions rightly leads to demands of tax parity with private pensions funded with post-tax dollars. More generally, the fact that Social Security taxes and Social Security benefits are treated differently under the tax code from contributions to and payments from private pension and insurance plans raises legitimate concerns about tax equity. For this reason, major changes in the tax treatment of Social Security benefits should be considered in the broader context of both overall retirement and overall tax policy.

Another question about Social Security's fairness is relevant here, indeed highlighted by the discussion of integrating tax and retirement policy. Many people have noticed Social Security's tax burden on low-income working families. "My God," someone said to us, "the less affluent pay more Social Security than income tax; it's crazy that I should pay the same proportion of my income to Social Security as the milkman." This decent concern reflects a partial misapprehension worth clarifying. It fails to take into consideration the progressive effects of the recently expanded earned income tax credit (EITC) on the tax obligations faced by low-income wage-earners with children.

The Tax Reform Act of 1986 set the level of the earned income credit at 14 percent of earnings up to $5,714, a level to be indexed for inflation. Starting in 1988, the credit operated, at lower percentages, on incomes up to $17,000, a figure that is also to be indexed. Only taxpayers with children are eligible for the credit, but it is "refundable." Workers with income tax liabilities less than their earned income tax credits receive a tax refund from the Internal Revenue Service (IRS). Workers with no tax liability receive the full amount of their EITC. The EITC is, in fact, a form of negative income tax.

Although generally not noted in discussions of Social Security, the effect of these changes is, as Joan and Merton Bernstein point out, "to cushion the impact of the FICA tax on millions of families with low and modest income."[34] What is confusing is that all of these families will still pay their FICA tax out of one pocket while receiving refunds into another. As tax policy, however, it means that very low income workers with children will receive nearly full offsets for Social Security taxes. At the same time, their continued payment of FICA taxes will maintain the link between work and benefits that precludes thinking of Social Security as simply another pot of public money.

In other words, when the joint effects of FICA and the EITC are understood, the burden of the Social Security tax at the lower end of the wage scale is not as great as it seems, at least not for taxpayers with children. Nevertheless, these arrangements could certainly be improved, in particular by extending eligibility for the EITC to all taxpayers and by increasing awareness of its availability. But here again, the "problems" to be solved are problems of overall tax policy and implementation, not the vagaries of a badly designed Social Security system.

Finally, if current demographic projections prove sound, we will certainly need to revisit the retirement age adjustments made in 1983. Indeed, it appears that changes in retirement practices are occurring that will require a rethinking both of the culturally appropriate retirement age and of the requirement that pensions be paid only to those engaging in no substantial paid work. Renewed efforts to integrate both the elderly and the disabled into the work force could easily reduce future demands on both disability and retirement pensions. And so it goes. Things change, and so must Social Security policy. But these social changes are gradual, and the responses they require from Social Security are both incremental and modest. That has been the history of the past fifty years and almost certainly will be the experience of the next seventy-five.

These sorts of reform proposals suggest some straightforward principles for adjustments to Social Security pensions. First, reformers must be very cautious. This is a program in which the magic of compound interest can produce big future effects from very small current adjustments. Second, issues of FICA tax equity cannot be divorced from more general questions of income tax equity and public policy toward private pensions. Third, and following from principles one and two, this is a system that demands calm advance planning to deal with both economic and demographic contingencies, not feverish manipulative response to one or another crisis. Happily, that has been the dominant tendency of Social Security policy-making, however overheated the popular political discourse.[35]

NEEDLESS WORRY AND SOCIAL INSECURITY

The problems Social Security has faced in recent decades have severely damaged public confidence that the system is soundly financed and competently managed. The young have experienced increasing doubts about their future benefits, and the old have felt their security attacked every time short-term insolvency seemed imminent or budget deficits prompted calls for benefit reductions. Every instance of economic turmoil brings Social Security back on the agenda of discussion, and each episode of Social Security–bashing brings tons of mail to the Congress attacking unjustified threats to the well-being of the aged. In the process, a seemingly prudent alarm has played a destructive role.

When macroeconomic events presented obvious difficulties, too many critics regarded Social Security as a culprit, not a victim. When our fiscal policies produced unprecedented deficits, too many doomsayers implicated Social Security, even though the system has lessened rather than increased our deficit problem. Worst of all, prudent adjustments have been saddled with excessive emotional freight. The rhetoric of crisis has too often been used to make required changes palatable. The cost of this practice has been very high. The changes introduced—even when adequate to the problem—have failed to lay to rest fiscal fears roused to panic proportions. And, when surpluses arise, the rhetoric of crisis returns. Indeed, it sometimes seems as though all of print journalism's computerized typesetting equipment has been invaded by a curmudgeonly hacker who instructs it to include the word "crisis" at least once in every paragraph in which the words "Social Security" also appear. In that sense, we have gotten less security from our prudent practices than we deserve.

The insidious and unnecessary atmosphere of crisis that has surrounded the process of Social Security reform in recent years has undermined confidence in our political capacities. If a crisis is declared every time even a modest adjustment in Social Security is needed, the cumulative effect is a corrosive sense that we cannot manage our collective affairs. Social Security, unlike many other institutions in American society, has been extraordinarily successful and has, by and large, been prudently managed. Still the myths of crisis continue to flow, inflaming those who oppose the system while rendering its defenders all the more resistent to adjustments of any type. The combination has been a bad political bargain. Competing charges and symbols clash in a sometimes stalemated game in which the political stakes are vastly disproportionate to the relevant policy alternatives. We have achieved diminished psychological security even as the provision of economic security has been maintained. This was not the promise of Social Security, and it should not be its future.

6

Misunderstanding Medical Care

If there is an arena of American social welfare policy in which the charges of undesirability, unaffordability, and ungovernability are persuasive, it is medical care. Claims of unaffordability are so pervasive that one need hardly be reminded of them. Whether it is the effect on government finances of rising Medicare and Medicaid expenditures or the annual reports that once again medical care inflation will far outstrip the general inflation rate in the economy, the threat to American competitiveness caused by dramatically increased health insurance premiums, or the risk of financial catastrophe faced by the uninsured, the message is always the same. The cost of medical care in America has become undeniably burdensome and promises to become more so.

The undesirability of our arrangements is also common fare in public debate. At the end of the 1980s we find between 30 and 50 million Americans who have no health insurance or are only minimally protected. Even those who are insured typically have gaps in their coverage that leave them on their own, or nearly so, in facing certain medical risks. What is worse, we pay more for this incomplete coverage than the citizens of other countries do for universal coverage. The United States spends over 11 percent of its GNP on medical care. Canada, France, and West Germany provide universal coverage to their populations at a cost of 8 to 9 percent of GNP. The United Kingdom, Japan, and Australia do it for between 6 and 7 percent of GNP. Given this state of affairs, our medical care arrangements provide easy targets for criticism on both moral and economic grounds. The richest country in the world, spending a larger share of its GNP on health than any other industrialized nation, should be able to do better.

The intractability, if not the ungovernability, of American medical care also provides grist for the commentators' mills. After all, what else could explain our dismal performance as compared with other countries? Whether the image is of American Medical Association (AMA) attacks on national health insurance, inept government attempts to regulate the supply of hospital beds, or the incapacity of the Congress to design an acceptable catastrophic care insurance package, most informed observers seem to agree that American medical arrangements have been, and currently are, out of control.

Although some of the dismal portraits of American medical care are overdrawn, we view these popular descriptions of a system in deep trouble as not very far from the truth. Serious problems undeniably exist in American medicine, and the direction of our most recent reform effort—cost control through private competition—is unlikely to make things substantially better. Some new form of restructuring is clearly required, but it is not obvious that our political institutions are up to the task.

The structure of American medicine has been the topic of nearly continuous struggle during the two decades that are the principal focus of this book. Major changes have occurred in both the politics and organization of American medical care, and the focus of public concern has shifted. A preoccupation with problems of access to care—symbolized in the 1960s by the establishment of Medicare, Medicaid, and neighborhood health clinics—gave way in the 1970s to a preoccupation with cost control. Now concerns about access are once again competing for attention.

The overwhelming focus on costs in the 1970s resulted from the rapid increase in both public and private health expenditures, combined with the general sense of economic insecurity that settled over the nation. We incurred larger and larger medical bills while our income stagnated. In the process, however, concerns about the effects of government controls in other regulatory arenas became confused with the problems of containing medical care costs. The convergence of these two trends produced in the 1970s a disposition to search for remedies for America's medical care ills in the wrong place—through increased enthusiasm for competition and privatization.

This competitive strategy has, however, failed to stem the tide of rising health expenditures, and its effect on the availability of medical care for the uninsured and underinsured can only be described as disastrous. As we shall see, international evidence suggests that the best way to deal with the access versus cost dilemma is through universal, governmentally organized health insurance. Until recently, such arrangements have been ideologically unacceptable to crucial actors in the political arena. But the 1990s may well be the decade in which economic facts and citizen preferences triumph over an increasingly costly and outmoded commitment to forms of medical provision and financing that are ill-suited to our current needs.

In medical care debates during the 1970s and 1980s, as in the struggles over Social Security and welfare provision, the ideology of privatism distorted sensible analysis. Critics whose major preoccupation was to reduce the state's role in welfare and retirement pensions can hardly be expected to see unified public financing as the solution to an increasingly critical set of medical care problems. Their influence helped keep the political agenda largely free of the very sorts of public initiatives that have worked well elsewhere. But, once again, this gets ahead

177

of the story. We must look back to see what happened to medical care provision and politics over the last two decades, before assessing where we stand as we enter the 1990s.

FROM ACCESS TO COST CONTROL: A PORTRAIT

Promoting Access. The preoccupation with the containment of costs is a relatively recent development in American health politics. Before the enactment of Medicare and Medicaid in 1965, the national government played a relatively modest role in the regulation of medicine and focused almost exclusively on broadening the access to and the supply of medical services and facilities. (To be sure, there had long been public provision of medical care through Veterans' Administration and Seamen's hospitals.) The federal government gave favorable tax treatment to community hospitals and directly subsidized hospital construction. The tax code also encouraged employer contributions to health insurance plans for employees. The dominant structure of American medical finance prior to 1965 was fee-for-service payment, with nongovernmental insurance (either Blue Cross/Blue Shield or commercial carriers) picking up a considerable portion of hospital and surgical costs and a much smaller proportion of nonsurgical physician fees and pharmaceutical expenses. The financing of care for the poor had three sources: the charity of community hospitals, payments by state and local welfare agencies, and the altruism of many physicians.

This system presumed that most people could pay for routine care and would be covered for large expenditures by employment-based health insurance. But this was never true for the population as a whole, and as medical care costs mounted, the problems for those not covered by employment-based plans became more serious. The Medicare and Medicaid legislation of 1965 sought to address this problem for the elderly and for those on public assistance. Although not universal, the 1965 legislation was a fundamental innovation. It put the federal government into the national medical care market for the first time as a major financier of medical services.

Medicare and Medicaid expenditures, combined with those for the military, veterans, and other smaller public programs, have made the federal, state, and local governments the largest purchasers of medical services. By 1989, government financed about 40 percent of total health expenditures (nearly 70 percent of that total through Medicare and Medicaid), whereas private insurance covered only about 32 percent. Patients paid the rest out of pocket.

The two decades since the 1966 beginnings of Medicare and Medicaid have been ones of extraordinary change and great confusion in the world of medicine. Its growing cost is one of the simplest indicators of massive alteration. In 1966, medical care accounted for 6 percent of America's GNP; in 1986, twenty years later, the figure was nearly 11 percent. Measured in dollars of constant purchasing power, total health spending nearly tripled between 1966 and 1986.[1] By any measure, medical care grew dramatically over this period—and it grew at an increasing rate. In real terms, the growth was more rapid in the 1980s than during what analysts had called the "health cost spiral years of the 1970s."[2] In such a context, shifts over very short periods are quite noticeable. In 1985, for example, Americans spent an average of $1,710 per capita on health care; two years later this figure was close to $2,000.[3] Expenditures for health care in 1990, estimated to reach nearly $650 billion, will represent almost 12 percent of GNP.[4]

In part, this dramatic rise in health spending is attributable to the fact that medical prices have increased faster than those of other goods and services. Between 1965 and 1986, the consumer price index increased 350 percent, but the medical care component of the index increased 484 percent. Although broadened access surely contributed to this price spiral, the trend cannot be blamed on Medicare and Medicaid. It was firmly established long before the establishment of those two programs. Indeed, the tendency for medical prices to rise more rapidly than other prices was greater before 1965 than it has been since. Between 1965 and 1986, medical prices rose at an average annual rate 38 percent above that of the consumer price index as a whole. Between 1950 and 1965, medical prices rose at an average annual rate more than double that of the consumer price index. Since 1950, medical prices have risen more slowly than overall consumer prices in only six years, five of which occurred after 1965.[5]

Unraveling the causes (and sequence) of the medical cost spiral is daunting in its complexity. Explaining the overall rise in health expenditures is even more difficult since factors other than differential medical inflation rates are involved. These include a growth in utilization rates and the increased complexity of care.

The spiraling cost of medical care—and the related alarm about the "crisis" in medical finance it has caused—is perhaps the one constant over the past two decades. In other ways the picture of American medicine has been more varied—a picture of both delight and dismay, of both fearfulness and hopefulness. Rapidly increasing costs have coincided with, although not necessarily caused, great improvements in health status and increased longevity since the enactment of Medicare and Medicaid in 1965. Indeed, after modest changes in morbidity and mortality rates during the period 1945–65, both infant mortality rates and life expectancy at age 65 rapidly improved. Infant mortality (measured as number of deaths per 1,000 live births) declined by more than half from 1960 to 1980, and four full years were added to life expectancy at birth during the same twenty-year period.[6]

A variety of factors—diet, exercise, the availability of new drugs, and surgical advances—contributed to a quite remarkable decrease in the age-adjusted death rates from one of the dread ailments of the 1960s, heart disease. Strokes, which with cancer and heart disease constitute the three components of the so-called deadly triangle of killers, declined sharply with the introduction of more effective drugs to reduce hypertension. Even automobile and other accidental deaths have moderated, partly in response to improved technology and better organization of trauma care. Only cancer resisted this surprising reversal. The war on it—fought with massive research and clinical expenditures in the 1970s and 1980s—has produced no dramatic breakthroughs, though the record of therapeutic improvement has been impressive for particular cancers, especially Hodgkins' disease, colon cancer, and some others.

Technological advances, often quite spectacular in their character and speed of diffusion, have given many Americans reason for optimism. The promise of medical miracles—the other side of the bargain for the great investment in medical research after the Second World War—seemed less fantasy than fact. The artificial heart became a tool—albeit a disputed and now disapproved one—where once it had seemed only a figment of science fiction. The development of the CAT scanner and, later, of magnetic resonance imaging transformed radiology and made the X-ray machine seem like a Model-T Ford.

There were, of course, darker features of the medical marvels.[7] Heart-lung machines made open-heart surgery possible, but respirators permitted vegetative patients to live on and on, raising financial and ethical quandaries for their doctors, nurses, insurance programs, and families. Darker still were the fears that medicine, for all its vaunted progress, not only was unable to affect many environmental threats, but was itself a source of danger. Concerns about "iatrogenic medicine" became a part of a significant health-oriented counterculture, if not of the mainstream of American life.[8]

In the mid-1960s, advances in therapy and the prospect of continuing medical improvement were all part of an optimistic vision of American health policy that included broadened access through Medicare and Medicaid. We were spending more for medical care, but we were getting more and better care. And we were getting richer. Then the bubble burst. Racial tension and urban unrest, the Vietnam War and its inflationary aftermath, the Arab oil embargo, "stagflation," and, in medical care, the explosion in costs—all contributed to a dismay that by the mid-1970s had us looking to the Great Society's programs, including Medicare and Medicaid, as sources of, rather than solutions to, our problems.

The increased focus on costs in the crisis language of the 1970s should not be taken to signal that the expenses of medicine had been largely ignored before. Rather, analysts had naively believed that expenditures would be contained in a more accessible world of medicine by paying hospitals only their "reasonable costs," doctors their "usual and customary" fees, and assuring, through utilization review committees, that expensive hospital care was really necessary. By the end of the 1960s, this optimistic incrementalism had given way to bolder plans for change.

The change in mood was apparent in the breadth of critical commentary about medicine and, simultaneously, in the willingness of politicians of every persuasion to consider forms of national health insurance. The recognition of trouble on the cost side was thus first linked to proposals that would, at the same time, broaden access. Senator Edward Kennedy's 1972 book, *In Critical Condition: The Crisis in America's Health Care,* symbolized both the shift in mood from optimism to dismay and the increased willingness to consider universal health insurance.[9] Although some favored universalism only as applied to catastrophic coverage, Kennedy proposed national health insurance, with the government acting something like a consumer cooperative in bargaining with organized medical providers about budget limits and proper charges. The Nixon administration countered with a plan for mandating health insurance at the workplace. The fierce debate on these and

182

other global proposals generated no overwhelming consensus in the period from 1970 to 1974. The Congress instead produced a series of less far-reaching changes in health planning and regulation. At the time, however, these "reforms" seemed preparatory to later action that would universalize health insurance coverage.[10]

As we enter the 1990s, the picture is very different. Few figures of political significance confidently promote government-financed, universal health insurance. The deficits of the Reagan years dominate political discourse and set severe limits on our political imagination. Intellectually, we live with the debris of the reform mentality of the 1970s and 1980s—a mentality that turned first to bureaucratic realignments as a means for "rationalizing" medical care provision and then, when those strategies seemed to fail, emphasized competition and privatization in a single-minded pursuit of cost control.[11]

Containing Costs. The institutional reforms of the 1970s were heralded with much fanfare, but they introduced a disjointed form of government regulation that was dispersed bureaucratically and disconnected from the major financing of care. With the usual advantages of hindsight, one can only wonder at the naïveté of these efforts to bring order to the mammoth and growing medical care industry. Health planning emerged in 1974, with 205 small agencies scattered around the country with the authority to say no to major capital expansion, but without a financial carrot to induce anyone to move in a different direction. The result was much debate, ending mostly in rushes to the state legislature or to the courts as providers sought protection from planning restraint.

Professional Standards Review Organizations (PSROs)—established by the federal government to monitor quality of care—were relegated in 1972 to a different set of agencies, dominated by physicians and disconnected in practice from the payments systems of Medicare, Medicaid, or the commercial and nonprofit health insurance plans. Medicare and Medicaid, once separate organizationally, were technically joined in what is now known as HCFA, the Health Care Financing Agency of the Department of Health and Human Services. But this new agency failed to unify Medicare and Medicaid administration, much less have an impact on health planning.

Throughout the 1970s, observers complained about the uneven distribution of care and the relatively high rates of inflation in medicine, but little was altered. The Carter administration supported serious legislation to contain hospital costs, but it was defeated in both 1978 and 1979 by a combination of hospital opposition, distrust of Carter's team, and more general skepticism about whether the federal government could accomplish what it promised. Inflation continued amid drivel about a "voluntary effort" to control costs by the health industry and the emergence of a new set of actors into much more important roles in American medicine.

Attracted by the gold mine of funds flowing through a system of retrospective, cost-based reimbursement, medical entrepreneurs came to see opportunity where the politicians had found causes for complaint.[12] In the hospital world itself, small chains of for-profit hospitals grew into large companies throughout the disappointing regulatory decade of the 1970s. The growth of HMOs (health maintenance organizations)—slower than promised by their supporters—came to include for-profit firms as well. Industrial giants like Baxter-Travenol and American Hospital Supply took their conventional dreams of increased market share and extended them through vertical and horizontal integration. A glut of physicians began practice, weakening the traditional power of doctors to control their terms of work.[13]

All of these changes in the structure of American medicine took place within the context of increasingly antiregulatory and anti-Washington rhetoric. Democrats and Republicans alike had been influenced by a generation of academic policy analysts—mostly economists—who ridiculed the costliness and captured quality of the decisions taken by supposedly independent regulatory agencies in Washington. The Civil Aeronautics Board and the airlines industry came to represent the distortions likely when government regulates any industry and, with time, the convention of describing any set of related activities with economic significance as an "industry" demythologized medicine as well. So even before the Reagan administration came into office the time was ripe for celebrating "competition" in medicine, getting government off the industry's back, and letting the fresh air of deregulation solve the problems of access, cost, and quality.

LIMITS OF THE COMPETITIVE STRATEGY

We should probably not be surprised that economists, looking at the health industry, would think that a good dose of private competition might be the answer to America's crisis in medicine. After all, the financing of medical care is dominated by large public payers, well-organized professionals, and highly regulated drug companies and insurers. This is not the free competition among atomized suppliers and purchasers that ideally would characterize a competitive market. Surely there is something to the notion that costs would come down if market distortions could be eliminated.

Moreover, the whole of medical provision is dominated by a "third-party payer" system in which the utilizer of care—the patient—faces only a fraction of the costs of that care at the time it is provided. For years economic commentators have blamed medical inflation on this type of financing. They point out that health insurance—private and public—pays for over 70 percent of the nation's medical bill. Thus, expensive as medical care is, patients, especially in hospitals, do not face the full financial consequences of their care. Widespread insurance insulates providers as well, especially those paid for each item of service.

185

Under such circumstances, there are strong incentives for physicians to recommend and for patients to accept that extra test or procedure, "just to make sure." This is what insurance experts call "moral hazard," in which the existence of insurance reimbursement encourages more spending than would otherwise take place.

This conception of health care's "distorted market" and health insurance's difficulties with moral hazard made medical care provision look ripe for reform in the direction of market competition. Indeed, this vision of reform largely dominated the debates over health policy in the late 1970s and early 1980s.

But to what degree can we assume that making American medicine more like a competitive market will solve our problems? The facts, as best we can know them, are not encouraging. The elimination of moral hazard in the insuring of modern medical care is all but impossible. No one supports the complete prohibition of health insurance—which legally removes the source of the "hazard." It is a classic case of a cure worse than the ailment. Americans undeniably want insurance protection from some or all of the medical expenses they face. What about the partial reduction of health insurance coverage by making patients—through increased deductibles and coinsurance—sensitive to the costs of most ordinary care? As a device to reduce moral hazard, private insurance companies have long used deductibles and coinsurance. But these measures obviously have not controlled the boom in medical spending nor have they been popular with the public.[14]

Other more acceptable "solutions" did in fact emerge in the 1970s. HMOs, strongly promoted by legislation in 1973, have obvious incentives to curb overutilization because they rely on fixed, annual premiums to finance care prospectively. Moreover, employers who foot some of the bill for medical insurance and government purchasers of care for the elderly and the indigent all have incentives to limit excessive services or fees. Throughout the 1970s, and increasingly in the 1980s, they tried to do just that. Indeed, one way to describe the period after 1975 is as a time of increasingly stringent constraints on the provision of care. Insurers have increased cost-sharing by patients and have imposed a host of restrictions on the use of popular and costly diagnostic and therapeutic procedures. As a result, physicians find themselves answering to more auditors of the appropriateness of their decisions than they ever dreamed possible. Employers have experimented with restrictions on which HMOs employees can choose for care, and they quite regularly limit reimbursement to an approved list of physicians who have agreed to negotiated fee schedules (preferred provider organizations, or PPOs). HMOs have imposed tighter controls on their physicians, as have hospitals under pressure from insurance companies, now much, much bolder about trying to "manage" as well as pay for care.

These efforts have had some limited success in constraining the health costs of particular firms, but not those of the nation. Competition disables controls as well as encouraging them. The cost containment efforts of group providers and employers are restrained by the ability of patients and employees to go elsewhere, either to other HMOs or to other employers who have more liberal policies. Insurers are limited by competition from other insurers who promise lower costs or less hassle. All payers must contend with the constant resistance of physicians and other health care professionals who sometimes evade the control systems or make threats to go elsewhere when controls are too stringent. Competition for patients, employees, and insurers thus constrains the degree to which suppliers can police strongly to avoid moral hazard. Moreover, much of this activity merely shifts rather than reduces costs.

The most successful strategy that has been devised for cost containment in recent years is hospital reimbursement by diagnosis-related groups (DRGs) rather than by payment for every expense incurred ("cost-based reimbursement"). The use of the DRG system, first for government payment by Medicare and then by some private insurers, has had some, but certainly not a dramatic, effect on cost escalation within hospitals. Note, however, that this is not a competitive strategy. It is nothing more, than government price controls made effective via monopsonistic market power rather than by direct legal constraint. And it turns out that costs saved as hospital expense mostly reemerge in the growth of outpatient care.

Nor does increasing provider competition among hospitals, doctors, testing laboratories, and drug companies seem to address much of the crisis in American medical care. The for-profit entrants into hospital provision have not been more efficient than their not-for-profit competitors, and no one thinks that the answer to cost containment is to build more hospitals of any type. Declining utilization is already threatening the continued existence of many hospitals.

If physician competition were the answer, it should already have worked. The stranglehold that the medical profession once had on the supply of new physicians has all but collapsed over the past two decades. Indeed, many now speak of a surplus of doctors, albeit one that is not well distributed either geographically or by medical specialty. Has the increased supply of doctors caused the price of doctor services to plummet? Hardly.[15] Indeed, the supply of doctors seems to create its own demand for services. Although contrary to economic theory, this feature of the medical care market is not surprising to patients. We all get most of our information about what health care we need from doctors. Given the potential efficacy of medical diagnostic and therapeutic techniques, the possibilities for increasing marginally useful interventions are almost limitless. Increased utilization of doctors and other medical providers is itself based on the advice of doctors. Such arrangements can accommodate an increased supply of doctors without having much effect on prices—or on health results.

The other major providers, testing laboratories and drug companies, already seem to operate in reasonably competitive markets. There have been some major advances in the efficiency of laboratory procedures that have substantially cut costs both for hospitals and for third-party payers. But it is not clear that there is much more progress to be made in this direction, or that any aspect of current public policy discourages such progress when technologically feasible. Similarly, public policy has already moved in the direction of increasing drug competition by breaking the control of physicians over prescription medication and allowing, sometimes requiring, pharmacists to substitute generic brands.

To be sure, the high profits earned by drug companies on new drugs during the patent period and the consolidation of drug companies in order to finance the costs of drug development limit competition in the pharmaceutical industry. It is unlikely, however, that our general patent policy will be (or should be) reversed, and there is certainly little public sentiment for relaxing the stringency of the FDA's safety and efficacy requirements in order to reduce the costs of drug development. To the degree that distortions in the pharmaceutical industry increase the cost of medical care, therefore, the problem is probably not solvable by greater doses of competition.

In short, it is very difficult to see how increased competition can resolve the problems of inflation in the medical care industry. Policies that would be "strong medicine" for economic distortions in the provision of care either are already in place, concern small portions of the overall medical care market, or have unacceptable side effects.

Equally important, the ratcheting up of private and public efforts to contain costs during the 1980s has begun to limit seriously the accessibility of medical care for those least able to afford it—the low-income, uninsured population dependent on hospital charity. Charity provision has been virtually eliminated in many hospitals, and attempts to avoid providing care to the uninsured have led to the spectacle of "patient dumping." Not only charity care, but also graduate medical education, technology development, and research are likely to be jeopardized as hospitals compete more fiercely on the cost-cutting side.

The same is true of insurance copayments and coverage limits. Many policies, including Medicare coverage, require patients to bear a percentage of the costs of their care and limit both overall benefits and payments for particular illnesses or procedures. Such restrictions have become increasingly popular with payers as costs have risen. The initial result of raising copayments or lowering reimbursement limits is simply a partial withdrawal of coverage. For many patients this may merely reinforce discretion and have no significant impact on access to needed care. For the most vulnerable, however, the sickest and the poorest, these restrictions inevitably result in less care or no care at all. And for the population as a whole these gross restrictions fail to distinguish between needed and unnecessary care.

The secondary effects of coverage limitations may be more widespread, if less dramatic. Reductions in primary policy coverage combined with fears of rising costs lead to the purchase of secondary insurance policies to fill in the gaps. "Medigap" policies to deal with Medicare copayments are but the most familiar of these arrangements. For those who can afford them, these policies greatly reduce the cost constraining effects of primary policy copayments or restrictions. Patients can obtain almost complete coverage. The insurance market thus reintroduces moral hazard while simultaneously increasing the administrative or transaction costs associated with multiple coverages—a topic to which we will shortly return.

As we enter the 1990s, the trend lines of "competitive" developments seem clear. The foundation for private financing of medical care—employment-based health insurance—is being eroded (and often abandoned). Employers say they cannot afford it and insurers claim they cannot make money on it. Instead, employers and insurers increasingly offer "managed care," by which they mean a comprehensive program of private regulation. Insurer-managers choose HMOs or restricted physician lists for the provision of care. They negotiate with physician groups and with hospitals on fees and costs and try to monitor most aspects of care to control unnecessary utilization. A world of medical care in which every physician decision concerning hospitalization must be "pre-certified" by a "managed care" business office and in which treatment for serious illness is closely supervised by an insurer-assigned nurse or social worker is the sort of world that most Americans with employer-based health coverage can expect if the trends of the 1980s continue.[16]

"HEALTH" VERSUS "MEDICAL CARE": A REVOLUTIONARY NONSOLUTION

Loss of interest in national health insurance has not been wholly a result of renewed faith in market mechanisms combined with a single-minded focus on cost containment. On the way through the economically tumultuous 1970s, the United States, like many Western democracies, discovered, or rediscovered, the differences between health and medical care. Drawn from a variety of sources, a new health consciousness greatly widened the considerations raised in discussions of health. Some commentators stressed the differences between well-being and what medical care expenditures actually purchased from doctors, nurses, and pharmacies. Others emphasized how change in one's way of life—diet, regular exercise, the management of stress, and so on—could improve not only how one felt but how one fared. Still others turned their attention to health threats that ordinary medical care simply could not prevent: slaughter on American highways, airborne pollutants endangering American lungs, foul water, accidents at work, and unemployment's corrosive effects on its victim's well-being. All of this was, in one sense, old hat, the message of nineteenth-century public health thinkers brought up to date.

The "new perspective on health"—to use the title of a 1974 report by the Canadian minister of health and welfare—implied some subordination of medical care as a source of improvement in the health status of developed countries,[17] but in most countries it did not entail ridicule of medicine. In the United States and in some other industrial nations, ridicule did arise as a logical extension of earlier repudiations of authority, assaults very much associated with challenges in the 1960s to university hierarchies, the political legitimacy of established officeholders, and conventional values. Ivan Illich was a leading exponent of the extended version of this new perspective—what later became known as medical nihilism.[18] Illich's message was twofold. Medicine could do little about the ills that really shaped the health status of most societies and, what was more, it could be dangerous itself. Talk shows, popular magazines, and newspapers took up this theme with a vengeance and, for a time at least, Americans heard of "iatrogenic medicine." By "iatrogenic" Illich meant the harm caused by medical treatment itself, the greater risk of infection within the hospital and the dangers of excessive intervention where simpler approaches were appropriate (caesarean versus natural births, for instance, or bottle versus breast feeding of the newborn).

Unlike other industrial democracies, however, only the United States (and Australia until 1975) did not have universal health insurance. As a result, the claims of medicine's limits (or dangers) affected American medical debates quite distinctively; the same arguments in our dissimilar environment had different implications. The central difference was this: Where universal access to medical care had, broadly speaking, been assured—in Britain, Canada, and Germany, for instance—the new perspective directed attention to more promising health promotion strategies. In the United States, however, the new perspective became for some another weapon to discredit national health insurance. If medical care was limited in its impact on health status, if the price of medical care was persistently rising faster than the rate of general inflation, then bypassing the controversial and costly development of national health insurance seemed to make sense. Why add lifeboats to the *Titanic* when a new direction might avoid major mishaps? If we had a proper *health* policy, we would not need national *sickness* insurance. This conclusion was less stated than suggested, less a formulation than a quiet inference from all the noise about medicine's troubles, limits, and dangers.

In countries where national health insurance (or its equivalent) was already in place, the politics of entrenched interests assured that personal medical care would not fall victim to the new emphasis on prevention. But, in the United States, the shift in policy attention contributed to the decline in sustained discussion of national health insurance in the period after 1975.[19]

The implications of the increased attention to health promotion are not yet settled as we enter the last decade of this century. On the one hand, there is a somewhat different cast—emphasizing healthiness—to much of health politics across the country. Smoking restrictions are at issue almost everywhere. States are addressing the safety of driving—whether the issue is seat-belt laws, the use of alcohol on the road, or speed limits. Environmental issues promise to occupy a prominent place on our political agenda in coming years. Public health education is also a source of controversy—most prominently highlighted by reaction to the AIDS epidemic.

The traditional politics of medicine, on the other hand, have not faded away. Scholars have documented the unlikelihood that preventive measures, in and of themselves, will sharply reduce American medical care expenditures.[20] Prevention can—and has—changed the incidence of disease, but, at best, it can only delay death and dying. Indeed, to the extent that American preventive practices have improved our health record—and there is good evidence that it has for heart disease and stroke—improvement has brought new issues of long-term care and frailty onto the agenda for health policy.

Prevention cannot avoid the financial consequences of care received nor make up for the results of care not given. The number of uninsured and underinsured Americans has grown sharply in the last decade, and many poor Americans lack even the most basic access to prenatal checkups and decent follow-up services for infants and mothers. Millions more live in fear of financial disaster from medical care that their health insurance will not cover. Expanding medical care delivery involves much more than seeking magic bullets of technical intervention. It is about justice as well as science. The extent to which norms of distributive justice are involved changes one's estimate of the significance of the new perspective on health. A right to health must include ready access to medical care when sick or fearful. That issue does not go away whatever the findings about the efficacy of prevention, the importance of the environment, or the wonders of changing to healthier ways of living.

For those nations that had satisfactorily dealt with issues of distributive justice in medicine, the "new perspective" was liberating. It provided guides to improving health without implying, as was sometimes the case in the United States, that improved access to medical care was beside the point. As a guide to what should be emphasized at the margin of future health policy, the new perspective was genuinely that, a new (and helpful) angle of vision on what to emphasize. But as a guide to the rationalization of medicine's access, quality, and cost, it was largely irrelevant in most countries and somewhat perverse in America. In a world of limited attention—and constant pressures on government and corporate budgets—the movement toward a more just system of medical care became a partial victim of the growth in enthusiasm for prevention. It is in this sense that the debate over medical care versus health in the United States has been singularly misleading and misguided.[21] It, like "competition," has failed to come to grips with the realities of medical care that America must address before the dawn of the next century.

AFFORDABILITY VERSUS ACCESSIBILITY

The crucial question for the 1990s and beyond is whether the double bind evident in American medicine can be made to yield to sensible and acceptable policy innovation. The constant talk about the financial crisis in America's medical industry and the persistent inaccessibility of medical care for a substantial number of Americans could, after all, describe either an inevitable economic condition or a straightforward political choice we have knowingly made. In either case handwringing would be a useless form of regret. It could represent a simple misunderstanding of the economic facts of life or, perhaps, a failure to face up to the necessary consequences of the medical arrangements that we, for other good reasons, have chosen.

The economic inevitability argument is straightforward. Americans, according to this line of reasoning, both believe in and benefit from a free market in goods and services. In such markets, prices allocate available supply and provide incentives for development of additional goods and services. In medical care, as elsewhere, there will be a substantial dispersion of prices representing quality differentials in the goods and services provided, and some consumers will be priced out of the market—or that part of the market which, cost aside, they would prefer. These are the ineluctable consequences of market provision. To rail against them is either to misunderstand or reject our economic system.

The argument from choice proceeds from this economic vision. Americans have not, after all, chosen market provision for all goods and services in all circumstances. But they have chosen to retain such provision in medical care, it is claimed, precisely because of the advantages of market allocation. Those supposed advantages include the continued freedom of "consumers" to choose their "providers" and, equally important, to discipline them by not choosing them. And so it follows that such a system, and no other, allows direct responsibility and accountability of physicians to their patients. In addition, the market provision of medical care creates strong incentives for the development of new technologies and procedures that, when exploited, benefit patients as well as providers. If we want to maintain these aspects of choice, accountability, and technological development, we must maintain something like our current medical arrangements.

To a degree, of course, these arguments are correct. No new arrangement for medical care provision will eliminate scarcity, only manage it in a different way. Every medical system must answer the question of access in more specific terms. The issue is not simply whether medical care is accessible. It is, instead, what care is accessible to whom, under what conditions, and with what effects? Nor does it seem likely that the huge financial rewards that flow to physicians can be removed without some effect on the character of medical care. The almost superhuman effort and commitment that we now expect from physicians may be a part of their professional ethic, but it is an ethic undergirded by a moral need to justify spectacular earnings. If cost containment means capping the market returns to physicians—and it almost certainly does—then we cannot expect such action to have no effect on how current physicians behave and who goes into the profession in the future.

Given these economic facts and the preference for medical arrangements that preserve both choice and responsibility, the cost-accessibility trade-off is real. How should we confront it?

One straightforward approach would attack the problem of access by universalizing health insurance through mandated, employer-based coverage with state-operated schemes for the unemployed. Payment for care would remain fee-for-service, but all payments (or virtually all) would be in third-party form. In all other respects, existing arrangements would be left intact. Such a "solution" would, of course, increase health costs by putting fifty million additional consumers firmly into the medical market.

It follows that in taking such action we would have to be prepared to increase both public budgets and the share of our GNP devoted to medical care. Perhaps we are willing to accept these consequences. We are a rich nation. Moreover, good health is a highly prized goal. If it costs 15 percent of GNP to have the sort of medical care we want, then perhaps we should simply pay for it and quit complaining. Spending more on medical care means giving up something else. But without good health everything else has less value.

Alternatively, we could accept the gaps in the current provision of medical care. After all, gaps in health insurance coverage are partly attributable to gaps in employment (or employment insurance). Instead of directing public policy toward medical care, perhaps we should emphasize labor market policies that will provide every American family with a living wage and access to employment-based health insurance. Moreover, to the extent that low income is associated with poor nutrition and high stress, attacking problems of poverty could improve health more than spending additional dollars on medical services. From this perspective, the current gaps in health insurance coverage are regrettable but do not necessarily call for a direct attack on the problem.

The gap-accepting approach might, indeed, be our only real option. Public acceptance of major increases in the national budget for medical care, both public and private, is hard to imagine unless supported by a more rapidly growing economic pie. But increased medical care spending could itself act as a barrier to improved economic performance. We are already in fairly serious trouble in terms of our global competitiveness, and adding 5 or 10 percent to labor costs would not help, no matter in whose budget—industry or government—the initial accounting entries appeared.

One might conclude from these arguments that in medical care, as elsewhere in the American welfare state, the claims of crisis and looming disaster are misdirected. We do have problems, but they result from our prior choices and commitments. Those choices are in no way sacrosanct, but they do have reasonable explanations. And, in any case, they are unlikely to be totally rejected. There is a real trade-off between accessibility and affordability, but it surely can be managed over the coming decades in the same incremental fashion as in the recent past. Those who subscribe to this view regard those who simultaneously seek more access and lower costs as simply misguided.

THE REAL WORLD INTRUDES

Although the foregoing may seem a hardheaded and realistic approach to American medical care, it is in fact neither. It exalts theory over empiricism, neglects the stated wishes of Americans with respect to medical care, and presumes the existence of choices that are rapidly disappearing. These are startling statements, perhaps, but the facts are increasingly difficult to deny.

Unlike other aspects of the American welfare state, our medical care arrangements are not now nor have they been in the recent past congruent with what Americans say they want. Virtually no American thinks it just for anyone to be denied necessary medical attention because of inability to pay. Both opinion polls and ordinary discourse confirm that an overwhelming majority of Americans view medical care as different from other goods and services. Beyond that, most Americans regard medical costs as unreasonably high. Indeed, objections to high costs and limited access have led the overwhelming majority of respondents in polls throughout the 1980s to agree that American medicine needs fundamental change. Clear majorities favor national health insurance financed by taxes and paying for most forms of care.[22] In contrast to our pension system, Americans do not have the health care system they say they want.

If what we have been claiming in these pages about the American welfare state's enduring commitments to social insurance and broadened opportunity is reasonably accurate, this should not come as a surprise. Both commitments are bolstered by universal access to medical services. The relevant political difference between our medical care policy and our pension and welfare policies is that for complicated but quite consistent reasons universal health insurance has always failed to surmount the entrenched opposition of multiple special-interest groups.

It is increasingly difficult to argue that the public's support of universal health insurance expresses merely an uninformed or self-indulgent regret. In virtually every other developed country, access to essential medical care is assured to the whole of the population. Moreover, as we noted earlier, universal provision everywhere else costs much less than partial provision in the United States. We spend roughly 3 percent more of our GNP on medical care than Canada, France, or West Germany, 5 percent more than Australia, Japan, and the United Kingdom—all countries with universal coverage. If the trade-off between cost and accessibility has not been wholly eliminated elsewhere, it surely has been rendered less poignant.

Perhaps the United States should expect to spend more, even while covering less. But this argument wears thin very rapidly. The argument is thin first because international experience indicates rather clearly that arrangements that produce universality also produce cost control. The comparison is particularly dramatic in Canada, where comprehensive health insurance went fully into effect in January 1971. At that point both Canada and the United States were spending roughly equal shares of their income on medical care. In addition, the two countries had experienced nearly identical patterns of escalating costs over the prior two decades, hardly surprising since the Canadian and U.S. medical markets were almost identically organized. Between 1970 and 1990, however, the amount of America's GNP devoted to medical care increased from 7.5 percent to approximately 11.5 percent. In Canada, by contrast, the increase was only from 7.5 percent to 8.5 percent (see figure 6.1).

The argument that the United States case is and can remain special also falters because it does not consider that these additional percentages of GNP devoted to medical care bear directly on the global competitiveness of our industries. American managers and workers are rapidly facing some very unattractive alternatives. In order to finance the escalating costs of health insurance, firms must either reduce the overall compensation of their employees by reducing medical coverage or substitute reductions elsewhere (in wages or other nonmedical benefits). In short, the high cost of American medical care will either cause us to lose markets, or it will cause American jobs to pay less well.

Simply put, our singular experience of continuously high rates of medical inflation is making us poorer. Indeed, it might not be too much to suggest, as a leading Canadian health economist has already done, that Americans' poor performance in allocating income to savings over the past twenty years is partly explained by our allocation of income to medical care.[23] If we must spend 3 to 5 percent more of our income on medical care than our contemporaries in France, West Germany, and Japan, not to mention the Commonwealth countries of Canada, the United Kingdom, and Australia, then it is perhaps not surprising that we have less of our income to allocate to savings.

Finally, the belief that we spend more to get more neglects the extraordinary inefficiencies of American medicine. In 1985, for example, the administrative costs of the American system—that is, the costs simply of handling the flow of paper and dol-

Figure 6.1: Total Health Expenditures, Canada and U.S., 1960–1987 (Percent of GNP)

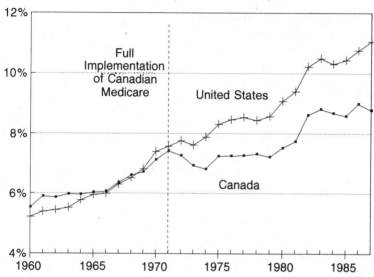

SOURCE: For the United States, Division of National Cost Estimates, Health Care Financing Administration. "National Health Expenditures, 1986–2000." *Health Care Financing Review,* 8:4 (1987), 1–35, and *Statistical Abstract of the United States,* yearly. For Canada, Health and Welfare Canada, "National Health Expenditures in Canada, 1975–1987" (Ottawa, Ont.: Health and Welfare Canada, 1987) and Canada, Department of Finance, "Economic Review," April 1985.

lars—were $95 per capita. In contrast, to administer their national health insurance system, Canadians paid only $21 (Canadian dollars) each. The extra bureaucratic expense of running our medical industry is estimated to account for nearly one-quarter of the overall difference in the costliness of American as opposed to Canadian medical care.[24] (See figure 6.2.)

Moreover, these estimates do not take into account the administrative costs that are extruded onto patients in the United

States. In the current climate, one in which every insurer and provider attempts to shift costs to someone else, dealing with medical insurance paperwork imposes enormous time and anxiety costs on consumers. Even those of us who are supposedly "fully covered" are anxious that coverage will be denied on the basis of unintelligible technicalities. This anxiety is coupled with the knowledge that, even if the denial is erroneous, as it often is, it will be an arduous and time-consuming process to correct the errors. Meanwhile, the mailboxes of the elderly and infirm collect increasingly threatening notices from computerized billing systems programmed to help medical providers and insurers shift costs to others and hound deadbeats, not to help consumers understand the terms of their mystifyingly complex coverage.

It is hardly surprising, then, that many Americans now ask themselves whether they must continue to have a medical care world characterized by uneven access, persistent inflation, inefficient administration, and high anxiety. Are these the inevitable prices we must pay for freedom of choice and high-quality care? Indeed, are we getting the high-quality care and freedom of choice for which we supposedly struck this bargain?

To answer the last question first, it seems clear that many Americans with ready access to the medical system regularly do get very high-quality care. It is less obvious, however, that this high-quality care has a significant impact on the public's health. Our morbidity and mortality rates are no better, and sometimes worse, than those of many countries with quite different arrangements that pay a much smaller share of their GNP for medical care. Although such gross data are only suggestive, it seems likely that Americans are paying a great deal for some combination of amenities in the provision of care and reassurance that they are healthy through the use of very expensive diagnostic technologies. It seems quite unlikely that shifting to arrangements satisfactory to the citizens of Canada, Australia, Germany, and Japan would make us less well.

Freedom of choice, the other major value to which we aspire, is hardly the dominant sense that most Americans have of their own access to medical care. And their impressions are not misleading. Group practice and specialization long ago eliminated most Americans' experience of the family doctor. To retain coverage and avoid large copayments, most Americans must choose physicians from approved lists and buy prescription drugs in the form and from the source specified by their medical care plans. We may choose a health insurance plan or an HMO, but nearly every other choice about our care is made by a bureaucratic provider or payer rather than by the patient.

In addition, as employers and insurers struggle to pare costs, they, of necessity, impose more constraints on the independence of physicians and hospitals. Increasingly physicians must sacrifice their own judgment about the utility of various diagnostic and therapeutic procedures to that of HMO, hospital, or insurance company managers. Insurance companies may have coined the term for this practice only recently, but "managed care" has already become the dominant reality for most of us. In other words, there is much reason to believe that we are getting the worst of both worlds—very little freedom of choice for either patients or providers combined with high costs and continuing anxiety about access.

THE EXAMPLE TO THE NORTH

Comparisons with other countries are often enlightening, but they seldom convince the skeptical that a foreign system, whatever its virtues, can be transplanted to American soil. The Canadian experience may be an exception to this general rule. With Canadians we share a common cultural heritage, increasingly integrated economies, and a tradition of constitutional federalism. Moreover, as we noted earlier, until Canada consolidated its national health insurance program in the early 1970s, Canadian and American styles of medical provision were nearly identical. If a different form of medical care financing can work well in Canada, it should also work reasonably well in the United States.

That it does work in Canada seems undeniable. Not only is coverage universal and cost containment much more effective than in the United States, but Canadians themselves are warmly attached to, rather than disaffected from, their medical care system. This attachment was demonstrated conclusively in the 1988 Canadian federal elections. The incumbent Progressive Conservative government ran on a platform that promised ratification of the free trade agreement with the United States. Although many Canadians were understandably concerned about further integration of their economy and culture with the United States, a substantial majority seemed to support the government's position. All was nearly lost for the Progressive Conservatives, however, when opposition parties began to argue that signing the agreement would lead to destruction of Canadian national health insurance. Almost overnight the Conservatives lost their lead in the opinion polls, with a swing of nearly 15 percent of the electorate. Only a concerted counter-campaign by the government to convince the electorate that there was no connection between free trade and government health insurance preserved the government's narrow victory, although with less than a majority of the popular vote.

To be sure, Canada's public health insurance—which they call Medicare—is not perfect. There is regular and fierce political controversy as provincial governments bargain with medical care providers about the terms under which care will be provided. But after nearly twenty years of operation, dire predictions that government control of medical care would lead to horrendous waiting times for services, a brain drain or undersupply of doctors, and loss of professional quality seem clearly false.

This is not the place for a full-blown description or discussion of Canadian Medicare. Its basic outline, however, is quite straightforward. The federal government conditionally promises each province that it will prepay a substantial portion (roughly 40 percent on average) of the costs of all necessary medical care. The federal grant is available as long as the province's program is *universal* (covering all citizens), *comprehensive* (covering all necessary hospital and medical care), *accessible* (no special limits or charges), *portable* (each province recognizes the others' coverage), and *publicly administered* (under control of a public, nonprofit organization). All ten provinces maintain health insurance plans satisfying these criteria. Each pays for the care provided by contracting separately with hospitals and doctors.

The practical dynamics of these systems are also simple, at least in outline. The hospitals' total budgets and physicians' fees for various services are determined annually in negotiations between provincial governments and the providers of care. As in the United States, most hospitals are public or nonprofit, and physicians practice in diverse individual and group settings. Unlike our current situation, the decisions of Canadian providers about care for particular cases are regulated only *ex post* by nongovernment professional groups. Patients choose their own doctors; doctors bill the province; hospitals work from global budgets, not itemized billings. Hassles over insurance claims, gaps in coverage, and bureaucratic incomprehensibility are, for practical purposes, nonexistent. The government health agency is the only payer in each province, and it constrains costs through the annual negotiations over hospital budgets and physician payments. Administrative costs are, as a consequence, negligible by American standards.[25]

There are many other interesting features of the Canadian system that would bear more extensive analysis. Patient, provider, and provincial incentives are, as to be expected, complex in practice.[26] Nevertheless, it does seem clear that most of the negative effects that economic theory might have predicted—

Figure 6.2:   Cost of Health Insurance Administration, Canada and U.S., 1960–87 (Percent of GNP)

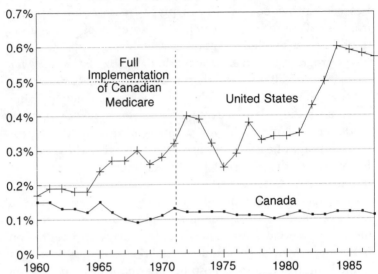

SOURCE: For the United States, Division of National Cost Estimates, Health Care Financing Administration. "National Health Expenditures, 1986–2000." *Health Care Financing Review,* 8:4 (1987), 1–35, and *Statistical Abstract of the United States,* yearly. For Canada, Health and Welfare Canada, "National Health Expenditures in Canada, 1975–1987" (Ottawa, Ont.: Health and Welfare Canada, 1987) and Canada, Department of Finance, "Economic Review," April 1985.

obvious rationing, long queues, worrisome physician flight, and technological obsolescence—have not emerged. There is, and has always been, some movement of highly trained, highly prized personnel from Canada to the United States. Physicians are no exception. But this trend was not greatly affected by Canadian national health insurance, and the numbers have always been small, never enough to offset a steady increase in the number of practicing physicians. Canada's physician-population ratio has been, and remains, comparable to that of the United States.

At the outset, the existing fee schedules of provincial medical associations were accepted, although in most provinces, payments were initially set somewhat below 100 percent to reflect the elimination of uncollected amounts. Since that time, changes in the structure and content of the schedules have been negotiated by provincial medical associations and ministries of health. The process of fee-setting is one of extended negotiation, not of unilateral imposition. Physicians were the highest-paid professionals in Canada prior to the introduction of universal medical insurance; they still are.

Canada does ration medical care. So does the United States and every other country in the world. We continue to ration by income, ability to pay, and geography. As a result, our access to care and the quality of that care vary enormously, and many experience long waiting lists and substandard facilities, if they get care at all. By contrast, Canada and most other countries in the developed world attempt to provide a more uniform standard of care to the entire population. Rationing is on the basis of relative medical need, largely determined by physician judgment.

At certain times and places there are substantial waiting lists for selected surgical procedures, but overall rates of hospital use per capita are substantially higher in Canada than in the United States. The vast majority of patients are cared for in a timely manner; long waiting lists reflect occasional managerial problems rather than chronic shortages of facilities. Priorities for care are determined by clinical judgments of relative need, not by bureaucratic rules, ability to pay, or arbitrary age restrictions.

On the other hand, certain high technology items are scarcer in Canada than in the United States. Canada provides access to a full range of high technology facilities, but there is significantly less abundance and little competition for market share. Expensive capital equipment is first approved only for tertiary care centers, and subsequent diffusion is closely controlled by provincial funding agencies. Although this control results in lower rates of utilization of some technologies in Canada—cardiac surgery, magnetic resonance imaging, and so on—this is not necessarily a bad thing. Throughout North America, there is serious concern about the appropriate use of new procedures. Inappropriate use is both financially costly and medically dangerous to patients.

The slower diffusion and more limited use of some new technologies could be viewed as evidence of lower-quality care. If quality is defined as easier access to high technology services regardless of appropriateness, then the American system offers higher-quality care. But this is a circular argument. If quality is defined in terms of health benefits rather than of service mix and levels, in terms of health results rather than of the dispersion of technology, then there is no evidence of a Canadian disadvantage. And if one of the relevant results is consumer satisfaction, then both polls and political behavior would put Canadian national health insurance well in the lead.

The generally high levels of Canadian satisfaction suggest the need to take account of the distributive dimension of health care quality. When quality is defined as the best technologies and facilities available to the most privileged members of a population, rather than as the facilities available to the average individual, American medical care ranks among the best in the world. But it is also true that some aspects of American medical care would be considered intolerable in other comparably advanced nations. Canada has fewer centers of technological excellence, but the average level of care is, by any definition, at least the equal of that in the United States.

Like the successes of our own welfare state, the generally high marks that Canadians give their own medical arrangements are sometimes lost in the rhetoric of political crisis. The nature of Canada's national health insurance is such that much of the bargaining for resources and control is carried out in the public arena. Provincial ministers of finance typically forecast imminent bankruptcy; medical associations threaten dire consequences as a result of chronic underfunding; and the media, always hungry for controversy, seize on the extremes of these positions. But the controversy that sells newspapers should not be interpreted as calling into question the fundamental principles that form the basis of Canadian Medicare.

The majority of Canadians place a very high value on their Medicare. It is widely viewed as Canada's greatest sociopolitical achievement and, as such, it is regarded by most Canadians as a sacred trust. No Canadian politician would dare advocate abandonment of the principle of universal access on equal terms and conditions. Canadian Medicare thus has political problems reminiscent of those we have associated with American Social Security pensions. If anything, politicians are invited to cling too tenaciously to the status quo. Those are problems to which, in medicine, the United States might easily aspire.[27]

GETTING THERE FROM HERE

Movement toward a more affordable and governable form of health care may be, almost certainly is, preferred by most Americans. But that is no assurance that we will achieve meaningful reforms. The politics of medical care in the United States has traditionally favored free market ideology. The preferences of providers and insurers have usually taken precedence over the lessons embedded in foreign experience and the disappointments of our current arrangements. Only a substantial change in politics as usual could produce major reform.

We are hardly sanguine that such reforms will be forthcoming in the near term. Nevertheless, there is cause for some optimism. One of the most hopeful signs is to see that paragon of made-in-America patriotism and shrewd marketing, Lee Iacocca, calling for national health insurance. In doing so he represents many large employers who see themselves increasingly threatened in international and domestic markets by the relentless inflation in medical care. The small business community is quickly catching up in complaint because the costs of health insurance are even more onerous for them. Eschewing the market and even its usual demand for state and local control, the American Chamber of Commerce called in 1989 for federal legislation that would ensure that small employers had insurance options at reasonable rates, free of exclusions and limits that severely restrict coverage. Employers large and small see a clear likelihood that they will soon be charged for mandated coverage, both for their own employees and for the unemployed, as states seek to cover the uninsured without raising taxes.[28]

Second, the opposition of private insurance companies to health insurance reform is decreasing. They are having great difficulty making money on medical insurance. The combination of inflation, costly technological development, and an aging population has put them on the wrong side of the cost curve. More important, consumer dissatisfaction is fueling demands for legislative action. The insurers are desperately looking for a solution that will bring insurance to the uninsured, stop the practice of "skimming" (fighting for the healthiest customers and ignoring or mistreating the less healthy) that is creating much of the consumer unrest, and yet leave insurance administration to the insurance companies rather than to the state. They fear that the reform options are rapidly shrinking to a choice between a universal, mandated private insurance program, with substantial regulation of terms and rates, and a state-run insurance scheme that eliminates private insurance.

Finally, physicians are increasingly aware that they cannot avoid regulation. Their behavior will be regulated either by hospitals, insurance companies, and government purchasers or by some more global arrangement that puts the whole of the medical care system under state management. As they look at Canada's Medicare, they are certain to be struck by the degree to which Canadian physicians bargain explicitly with payers over the terms and conditions of payment for care, and the degree to which those bargains leave the day-to-day decisions about medical care to professional judgment. Although Canada has socialized health insurance, the freedom of Canadian doctors from bureaucratic restraints in the practice of medicine almost certainly exceeds that of their American counterparts.

There are the makings of a compromise here. The public wants broadened and simplified coverage at reasonable cost. Firms want to reduce the costs of covering their employees and, certainly, to avoid paying for the costs of the unemployed. Insurers know that they are in a new ball game in which at best they will be administrators of managed care and at worst they may be excluded from the market. Perhaps they could manage everyone's care on behalf of state insurance schemes. In short, although movement toward something like the Canadian system may appear ideologically a large step, in practice most of the pieces needed for a state insurance scheme are already in place, and interest-group politics might join with popular sentiment to permit such a move.

Yet, even with these developments, there are major obstacles to the rationalization of American medical care. Although we almost certainly could reduce per capita costs while universalizing care, such arrangements would require that medical expenditures now divided among the government, employers, private insurance companies, and consumers be converted into public budget items. American politicians would have to be willing to put aside their fixation with where costs are counted and deal with real issues of public economies. In addition, the complaints of pro-competition, pro-market commentators would have to be ignored or rejected. Ideology would have to be countered with pragmatics, illusion with fact; and all this would have to be done by politicians who have been elected by running against government, against tax increases, and for the market.

The message conveyed to the American public since 1975— that less government is the key to controlling medical costs— must somehow be revised. It should be clear that the perceived trade-off between accessibility and cost in American health politics offers a false choice that is largely detached from the realities of medical care. In this corner of the American welfare state, the most pressing problems are ones of uneven provision and the absence of unified public control.

Marketing this revised message is not impossible, but it will take a form of entrepreneurial political leadership in domestic affairs that is always in short supply. Not only the public but also the makers of health policy will have to be persuaded that the key to achieving increased efficiency, reduced costs, and enhanced national competitiveness lies not in the removal of government from our medical care arrangements but in the opposite direction, in the adoption of a system of publicly financed, universal health insurance, an arrangement the public increasingly says it wants.

7

How Not to Think about the American Welfare State

Much of this book has been about misinformation. A quite re-markable proportion of what is written and spoken about social welfare policy in the United States is, to put it charitably, mis-taken. These mistakes are repeated by popular media addicted to the current and the quotable. Misconceptions thus insinuate themselves into the national consciousness; they can easily become the conventional wisdom.

That many, if not most, Americans walk around with vague, misleading, and mistaken ideas in their heads about the Ameri-can welfare state is not necessarily a problem. Program admin-istration is in the hands of specialists who know better. Even the legislators who sometimes publicize and promote error are sel-dom themselves misled. And the academic commentators who provide much of the knowledge base on which policies are built and evaluated are properly skeptical of almost everything. So what is the harm? The harms are multiple. We will mention but two general categories.

First, there is a clear harm to democratic governance. If gov-erning elites know that people generally have mistaken ideas about the welfare state, they can react in one of three ways: They can try to change the conventional wisdom; they can govern as if the conventional wisdom were true; or they can

213

speak in terms that reflect popular understanding but attempt to govern on the basis of their quite different conception of the facts. The first alternative is seldom chosen. Few things are riskier to political tenure than an attempt to market new ideas. Happily, most politicians also reject the second option. But that exercise in political responsibility leaves dissembling as the only path available to policy reform combined with political success. This is political leadership built on the twin pillars of fear of, and contempt for, public opinion. And that is hardly anyone's ideal of a well-ordered representative democracy.

Disordered democracy does not, however, leave political elites free to follow their own principles or prejudices. The gap between elite and popular understanding constrains the possibilities for policy development. If reform must be marketed in terms of dominant misconceptions, certain things are both unthinkable and undoable. Language, even political language, is not "infinitely" malleable, and "the people" are not fools.

The second harm of mistaken ideas, then, is that they can lead to mistaken policies. If legislators must always act as if public welfare were an evil, luring the poor into dependency, destroying family values, and generating an ever-growing underclass, then the only successful reform would be one that caused both welfare and the poor to disappear. And if that is the case, then it is extremely difficult to develop and sustain programs for deprived populations, programs that, by their very nature, can have only limited success. Everything that is tried must be a failure. And every new "reform" must be marketed, and at least partially structured, in terms that assure its eventual failure as well.

The political dynamics of guaranteed failure thus also virtually ensure poor administrative performance in the periods between policy shifts. If welfare programs are by definition an arena of political failure and programmatic instability, the "best and brightest" will seldom be attracted to welfare administration. And even those who try will find it impossible to manage

214

vast systems that are constantly said to be failing and on the verge of being scrapped. It is hardly surprising that the hardy altruists who do make a career of welfare administration soon redefine their goal as survival rather than success. The politics of welfare tends to make the professional lives of the public administrators of welfare almost as marginal as the lives of the clients whom they try to serve.

Or, to take another example: The fiscal difficulties of medical programs are regularly interpreted as the result of inadequate competition in the health industry. There is surely something to this view. But that does not mean the problems of health costs can be moderated by trying to make the health market look like the market for pork bellies. Indeed, it seems clear that solutions lie in quite the opposite direction—in consolidating buyers and sellers into groups that can exercise effective countervailing power. Because these sorts of solutions cannot sensibly be portrayed as making medical care more competitive, they can only with great difficulty be made a part of medical policy discourse.

More particularized misunderstandings also affect our range of choice with respect to particular issues. We confuse "target efficiency" with programmatic effectiveness and, ironically, lament the failure of our most successful antipoverty program, Social Security pensions, to address the poverty problem. We eschew income support for the "deserving poor" in order to avoid the dependency of the "undeserving" with little appreciation of how the availability of income support actually affects work effort or family formation. In short, the general level of misinformation about the American welfare state is not without great cost.

But what is to be done? After all, the American public is not going to be converted overnight from sports fans into policy analysts. The information needed to understand American social welfare policy and to evaluate proposed reforms critically is enormous. No substantial body of citizens is likely to pay the costs of becoming and remaining well-informed on these issues. And, as we must readily admit, the problem of public understanding is not entirely a problem of unavailable information. Public commentary is a mix of appalling ignorance and cogent, sometimes highly insightful, analysis. If misconception seems often to inhabit the public consciousness, it may simply be that certain ideas are more hospitable than others. People believe what they want to believe, and no amount of haranguing by well-intentioned fact-grubbers is likely to change their minds.

Perhaps. But as we said at the beginning of this book, we are not ready yet to throw in the towel. As we have thought about these issues, it has occurred to us that we are not necessarily dealing with a set of disparate factual errors. Instead there seem to be common patterns in the analysis of social welfare issues that lead to different, but methodologically related, misconceptions. We have, therefore, capitalized these common threads into a set of rules about policy talk. Here are the rules, along with some illustrations of the errors engendered by a failure to heed them.

RULE 1: PROJECTIONS ARE NOT FORECASTS

Much of the talk of crisis in the welfare state or in social welfare policy involves a very simple technique—the projection of current trends into the future. This is a splendid way to produce fright but a poor way to forecast the future. Using this technique, consider the terrible fate of your four-year-old. For the last four years she probably grew at a rate of over four inches per year. At that rate, by the time she's twenty-one she will be ten feet tall!

But wait a minute, you might say. My daughter's growth is not like the growth of social programs or the economy or teenage pregnancy. Growth has natural limits, a natural stopping place. Social and economic processes do not. Well, maybe. At least we don't *know* that they do. And this difference is crucial to understanding both why projections are convincing and why they should not be.

First, recognize that while you are pretty confident that your daughter will not be ten feet tall, you don't actually know why she won't. You just observe that the adults you see around you were once rapidly growing four-year-olds and that they are not now giants. They grew quickly for a while, slowed down, maybe had another high-growth spurt in their teens, and then stopped growing. Moreover, if you looked carefully at individual growth rates you would find a lot of variability. Some achieved their full height by thirteen or fourteen; other late bloomers added an inch or two in their early twenties. Some grew pretty steadily, others in fits and starts. Much of this variability, as well as ulti-mate individual stopping places, was quite unpredictable. But everyone has enough experience with human physical develop-ment to presume that these background facts should be relied on rather than the projection of some current trend into the future.

Now think about trends in social or economic development. Presumably everyone is reasonably skeptical about economic forecasting. The projected growth rate for the next three months is not sufficiently reliable that any sensible person would stake much of their wealth on its accuracy. Indeed, there is no "it." The government has several forecasts, and private firms and individuals provide a host of others. They always disagree. If we extend such forecasts out a few years rather than a few months, they are surely fairy tales.

Yet look how often these tales are believed when talk turns to planning for the future. We have had relatively flat median family income for the past fifteen years, so we will have the same thing well into the twenty-first century, notwithstanding steady and sometimes rapid income growth during the thirty years prior to 1973. We recently have had low fertility rates, so that will continue too, as presumably will the rate of medical inflation, the growth of social welfare spending, and the rising ratio of illegitimate to legitimate births. In fact, of course, we have little idea whether these trends will continue and, if so, whether at an increasing or a decreasing rate. Indeed, all such trends may have "natural" limits, but because the mechanisms of social change are poorly understood, we do not know how to predict when or where those limits will be reached.

Hence, we extrapolate into the future holding certain aspects of the present constant, even if by constant we mean a constant rate of change. We confuse the data on which this constant is based with what is usual, normal, or natural. We really have little choice. We should have a much healthier skepticism about these tales of the future. To the extent that they are tales of future dread or future delight, they probably say more about the personality of the forecaster than about the likely state of the world.

That same skepticism obviously applies as well to the tales your present authors like to tell. We have happily reported trillion-dollar buildups in the Social Security trust funds, for example, on the basis of the intermediate projections of the Social Security trustees. But what kind of "forecast" are we relying on here? The answer is not very inspiring.

The Social Security trustees are required by statute to make projections seventy-five years into the future—that is, to say what 1989 would be like from the vantage point of 1914. In part because they know this task to be preposterous, they make three projections—optimistic, pessimistic, and intermediate—using different average rates of change in the relevant variables (population, wage rates, mortality rates, etc.). Because no one has any good reason to be either optimistic or pessimistic about the state of the economy and the Social Security trust funds in the year 2050, analysts like us usually talk in terms of the intermediate prediction. That is thought to be more reasonable. But this is reasonableness of a very peculiar order—it takes as true a midpoint between predictions that one has no good reason either to accept or to reject. Mathematically there is no better strategy, but that does not make the prediction a good one.

Beware of projections masquerading as forecasts! Whenever a social policy analyst says, "At this rate . . .," start asking questions about why that rate should continue. And when people start projecting consequences more than five years down the road, you are probably justified in concluding that they are indulging a taste for science fiction.

RULE 2: INCENTIVES ARE NOT BEHAVIORS

Economists have become the policy gurus of the late twentieth century. We turn to them, or their methods, to predict the likely outcome of most changes in social welfare policy. Their stock in trade is a simple story. People behave rationally. If you increase or decrease the economic rewards of particular activities, you will get more or less of those activities, *unless,* of course, something else happens simultaneously to alter behavior in a different direction. Although simple, this story is also powerful. It makes perfect sense in terms of much of our ordinary experience and it allows fairly good statistical predictions regarding certain economic markets—at least in the near term.

The problem with the economists' story is really that it is too powerful or, at least, too convincing. People tend to forget both the "unless" qualification on the end of it and that nothing yet has been said about how much more or less we should expect. As a consequence, it is too easy to predict policy successes and policy failures that will never materialize. Moreover, as the social context of the story moves away from more straightforward economic applications, the calculation of advantage and disadvantage becomes increasingly complex. In the extreme, disincentives might be perceived as incentives, thus reversing the expected direction of change.

Consider a few of the examples that we have encountered in

219

the preceding pages. First, remember Harold and Phyllis. Charles Murray told a simple and superficially convincing story. Welfare did seem to be changing in a direction that provided greater incentives for avoiding marriage and for having illegitimate children. And we were, for a time, experiencing declining marriage rates, rising illegitimacy rates, and rising AFDC rates. It was easy to conclude that the changes in economic incentives—AFDC benefits—were driving the behavioral changes—illegitimacy and welfare dependency. But a careful look at the periods involved, as well as at the differential rates of change in different localities, revealed the hypothesis to be false. Incentives did not translate directly into behaviors—indeed, could not be shown to be affecting behavior at all.

The reason for the lack of correlation seems apparent. Decisions about childbearing, marriage, and living arrangements are very complex. They surely are not unaffected by economic incentives, but they are affected by a host of other factors as well. If those other factors—for example, the general societal perception of out-of-wedlock births or of single parenting—are also shifting, they may dwarf the effects of the economic incentives. And, even if they are not, there may be very few people for whom small changes in economic well-being would make a difference sufficient for them to change their sexual behavior or basic living arrangements. Reducing the economic price of illegitimacy has a much less predictable effect on behavior than reducing the price of bananas.

In addition, the economic incentives relevant to the issues addressed by Murray are themselves both more varied and more complex than his simple story suggests. It is the strength but also the vice of economic analysis to focus on isolated, easily measured economic variables. In the real world, the multiple pressures and diffuse expectations created by economic forces are much harder to sort out. Whatever effect changes in AFDC eligibility and benefit formulas have had on the behavior of the poor, a host of other economic factors—especially labor market conditions—have probably played a more important role.

Remember as well the story of Social Security and the savings rate. The straightforward suggestion was that the promise of Social Security would reduce the amount that people saved for old age, thereby reducing national savings and inhibiting economic growth. Since no one is willing to use this argument to attempt to repeal Social Security without even asking how much, that question was asked in a serious and sustained way. The results were quite surprising. Studies demonstrated that Social Security has positive, negative, and no effects on savings. That some investigators got positive effects led to a deeper puzzle. Could the basic incentive story be wrong? Perhaps people saw Social Security as protecting them from the demands of the improvident elderly so that saving for individual retirement became more attractive. On this interpretation, Social Security provided incentives rather than disincentives to save.

Indeed, a variant on the latter story is told by life insurance experts. The insurance industry opposed Social Security pensions and survivors' insurance precisely because the programs would limit the demand for privately funded annuities and life insurance. In fact, the reverse seemed to occur. Rather than merely altering the marginal demand for life insurance products, Social Security transformed the context within which such products were sold. Social Security actually provided life insurance sales staffs with a new marketing technique. First, it allowed them to provide a service. They got a foot in the door by offering to explain to a potential client exactly what their Social Security benefits would be. Second, having demonstrated that the client is, through Social Security, already planning for retirement or premature death (and after 1960, disability as well), the salespeople could then explain the gap between that planning and what the family really needed, a gap that could, of course, be filled by private insurance. Moreover, because the availability of Social Security benefits meant that the gap between resources and needs was smaller than it otherwise would have been, it seemed more feasible to many people actually to do something about it. They therefore bought more insurance, not less.

We do not offer this life insurance story, of course, for its general validity. It is based entirely on anecdotal evidence. But it nevertheless illustrates the extraordinary complexity of relating incentives to behaviors in particular contexts. Not only are there many confounding factors, but people also may interpret what has happened very differently than we would have imagined.[1] The world is not so simple: Incentives are not behaviors.

RULE 3: PURPOSES ARE NEVER UNITARY

In the preceding pages we have often chastised critics for the mistaken assumption that social welfare programs are designed to pursue a single purpose and are "failures" to the degree that they fail to achieve that purpose, fail to achieve it at least cost, or fail to pursue other purposes as well. This analytic genre is so common that it even has recognizable species. One of our favorites is the "Basic Contradiction Thesis." This thesis almost always takes the same form. First, the analyst notes that public programs in a particular policy domain have multiple purposes. Second, he or she notes that not all of their purposes can be achieved simultaneously. Third, the analyst points out that one or more of the programs under discussion is failing to live up to its stated goals or aspirations (a statement that is, of course, always true of every program). Next, the gap between aspiration and accomplishment is ascribed to the basic (or inherent, or fundamental) contradiction in the programmatic goals that have been chosen. Finally, there is a call for a unified vision that will permit us to cure the defects in existing policies.

A good example of the basic contradiction thesis is stated quite early in an otherwise excellent book on disability policy:

When disability policy is viewed whole, a fundamental contradiction appears. Simply put, this nation spends most of the money allocated to disability on programs that provide the handicapped tickets out of the labor force. At the same time, policymakers fund training programs and pass civil rights laws as an inducement for the handicapped to enter the labor force. Because disability has been subsumed under so many different headings, the contradiction goes largely unnoticed.[2]

As is customary with contradiction analyses, this one finds other anomalies in the programs under review. For example, the existing programs' use of at least three different definitions of disability or handicap is seen as a barrier to "a more rational disability policy." And there are, of course, contradictions within individual programs themselves. The persistently high level of legal dispute over workers' compensation awards contradicts a basic purpose of that program, to reduce litigation. The Social Security disability program retains its strange administrative arrangement, adjudication almost wholly by state agencies, in the face of an obvious desire to establish a national program of income maintenance. Vocational rehabilitation programs only reluctantly attempt to rehabilitate those most in need of their services. And so on.

We certainly would not claim that the programs under discussion are without flaws, indeed serious ones. Nor would we deny that some of those problems may be the result of contradictory features or tendencies within or among programs. The point is only this: To call attention to the contradictions in policies does not, by itself, make a major contribution to either policy analysis or political reform. All programs are compromises. Hence, all programs contain contradictions. Moreover, these contradictions are not accidental. They respond to sets of political preferences. Unless those political preferences have changed, to point out a contradiction is not to point out a mistake that will lead political actors to do better next time around.

We do not want to take on the burden of arguing that such critiques are never sensible. Sometimes they point to features of programs that should be further investigated and, perhaps, reformed. Our point is that because claims of contradiction are always correct, they are not generally very useful. And if the critic simply stops, rests his or her case after demonstrating the diffuseness or incoherence of programmatic purposes, the criticism is simply a tautology. Social purposes are never unitary and they are often—we are tempted to say always—contradictory. These multiple and often competing purposes are embodied in our collective efforts to address social welfare problems. To point this out, therefore, is not to distinguish good programs from bad ones. Indeed, such statements are both tautological and banal.

It is hard to overstate the ubiquity of the unitary purpose fallacy. Remember, for example, the critique of Social Security pensions that charges them with squandering social resources by making payments to the nonpoor. Or the overall critique of means-tested programs that they fail to "close the poverty gap." As we saw in those prior discussions, such claims are as myopic as they are ubiquitous. They simply fail to recognize that programmatic purposes are multiple.

A more charitable interpretation of these myopic critiques might be, of course, that the critic means to argue that we should have only one purpose, such as poverty reduction, or that one purpose should so dominate the values of the particular program that all other purposes are secondary, and distantly so. Abstractly considered, this is a more plausible claim, but it is still not very sensible. To see that this is true, let us consider the possible construction of the most straightforward sort of poverty reduction program—a negative income tax (NIT).

If a negative income tax is to have as its dominant, if not exclusive, purpose the relief of poverty, then the poverty line should be the income floor. Everyone should receive a transfer representing the difference between their annual income and the poverty-level income. If there is no difference, they get nothing. If they have no income, they get a payment equal to the poverty-level income for their family size and location. Between these extremes, earned dollars substitute one-for-one for government transfers. So far so good. This is a program that will eliminate all income poverty and waste not a cent on payments to the nonpoor.

But this is also a highly problematic program from several points of view. For example, this is a program that makes no moral distinction between people who work full time at low-wage jobs that fail to produce an income above poverty and people who do not work at all or do not try to work. We want each to have the same income. But, of course, American society is not morally indifferent as between these types of behavior—far from it. If the negative income tax is to have any chance of passage, it must reflect the real differentiation that we make between working and not working. Those who work should realize something for their effort. They should not, in effect, be taxed 100 percent on their earned income by the withholding of one NIT dollar for every dollar they earn up to the poverty level.

How can this be done? There is no way without compromising the NIT's antipoverty purpose. The simplest device within a negative tax scheme is to alter the implicit tax rate on earned income. What should that rate be? The standard approach is to ask what we consider a fair rate of tax on low-level incomes in the ordinary income tax system. That percentage can then be the amount by which negative taxes are reduced when there is earned income. The mathematics of this exercise, however, produce some surprising results. Assume, for example, that the poverty-level income for a family of three is $10,000 and that the basic tax rate on lower levels of earned income is 25 percent. If that tax rate were applied to negative taxes, payments would be made to any family with earned income of less than $40,000!

If we structure the negative tax program in this way, of course, we have made a major compromise with our antipoverty objective. We are not just failing to target the program exclusively on the poor; most of its beneficiaries will be non-poor. $40,000 is well above the median family income. Moreover, as we begin to think about the implementation of this program, we will discover that its effects suggest another purpose that has never loomed very large in American social welfare discussions. In order to finance such a program, positive taxes on incomes above $40,000 would have to be steeply progressive. The program would, in effect, be radically egalitarian. It would level incomes dramatically and, for many, painfully. This, combined with the facts that it would have staggering budgetary consequences and would make more than half the population welfare recipients, is certain to make our hypothetical NIT proposal a political nonstarter.

So, what can be done? Any number of things, but all will compromise the NIT's antipoverty goal in one way or another, and perhaps its other goals as well. We can, for example, reduce the baseline payment to those who have no earned income, so that those who work at low wages full time will always be better off than those who receive only negative tax payments. If we combine that with a very steep "tax" on earnings (the rate at which earned dollars substitute for transfer dollars), those who work full time will always be better off than those who work only part time and receive negative payments. Both approaches will, however, prevent the program from filling the poverty gap. The second will also entail unfair taxes on low-wage workers. Hence, from either value perspective—poverty elimination or supporting the work ethic—the program will be a failure.

There are, of course, other alternatives we could devise. We could be more generous, for example, filling the whole poverty gap, but only for special groups for whom work is not a realistic or approved option—the aged, the blind, the disabled, and children. But were we to do this, as we have in fact already done to some degree, we will necessarily fail again to fill the poverty gap for those we leave out of an approved category. Moreover, we will very likely begin to wonder whether poverty-gap-filling is what support of these categorical groups really ought to be about. Are we not also interested in helping the aged and handicapped maintain their dignity and standard of living? And, if so, is a means test that limits payments to the poverty-stricken consistent with that goal?

And so it goes. Wherever we turn complexity intrudes. This is not, we hasten to add, because as a society we are weak-willed and stupid, unable to define clear goals and stick to them. Complexity intrudes rather because it would be dumb to forget that we have more than one purpose and monomaniacal to structure public programs as if we did not.

Indeed, apparently unitary purposes are often really multiple and at least potentially contradictory. This is surely the case with poverty reduction. We do want to alleviate current income poverty. We also want to help people avoid becoming poor. This is the crucial insight contained in Charles Murray's notion of latent poverty. As a society, we are concerned not only about who is now poor but also with who would be poor but for public transfers, and why. Other things equal, we would rather eliminate poverty without spending money for transfer programs. If we can attack causes rather than conditions, then perhaps someday transfers could come to an end (or be reduced, or at least not grow). Moreover, Americans really do believe that to be self-supporting is to be better off—to have greater self-respect, confidence, and identification with one's community—than to receive welfare, even if one's income, whether from work or welfare, is identical.

Our antipoverty programs consequently want to address at least two antipoverty purposes simultaneously—the alleviation of current and the prevention of future poverty. But, as Murray also observes, these aims are potentially inconsistent. Current benefits reward existing conditions that, because rewarded, may persist. Murray goes on, of course, to build most of his argument on this difficulty and to conclude that only the elimination of all welfare could possibly eliminate poverty. As we have pointed out, this argument is deeply flawed. But its flaw lies in its failure to remember that incentives are not behaviors, not in its recognition of the necessarily compromised nature of social programs. Purposes are always multiple, and in a world of scarce resources, different purposes will at least compete, if not conflict. Beware of any argument that evaluates a social welfare program from a single perspective.

RULE 4: COMPREHENSIVE REFORM IS USUALLY NOT ON THE AGENDA

The language of reform needs reforming. Our programs are never "modified" or "adjusted." They are "overhauled," "revamped," "replaced," or "totally reconstituted." This is hardly surprising, of course. If the need for change is presented in terms such as "mess," "disaster," "failure," or "bankruptcy," then nothing short of a fresh programmatic start could possibly suffice to solve the problem. We are thus, to credit this rhetoric, perpetually in the throes of one or another major reorientation of the American welfare state. No one stops to ask how we as a people can assimilate a social welfare policy revolution every four or five years any more than we recoil from the claims of each automobile manufacturer to give us a totally new product every model year. We expect this inflated rhetoric and discount it accordingly.

Or do we? As citizens, most of us do not follow the details of social welfare programs. And even if we tried to do so, we would not find them as easily followed as the general path of automobile model changes. Hence, we are probably more susceptible to the claims of comprehensive reform in social welfare programs than we are to the assertions of newness that leap at us persistently from every form of commercial advertising. And, of course, to the extent that we are fooled by the political rhetoric surrounding social welfare reform efforts, we will be disappointed to learn, just a few short years hence, that total reform has had to be undertaken yet again.

Moreover, the rhetoric of comprehensive reform of welfare, pensions, medical care, or other social programs, because tied to the rhetoric of total failure, provides a quite different vision of social welfare policy adjustment than the advertising of "new features" does for automotive design change. The latter merely heralds improvements. Manufacturers do not begin their campaign for new fuel-injected engines by reminding us how crummy their old carburetors were. They do not focus our attention on solid-state ignitions with a long rehearsal of the ills of traditional automotive electronics. With automobiles our sense is of steady progress, not, as is the case with social welfare policy, of cycles of failure and reform.

As we have previously rehearsed, we do not think that these rhetorical excesses have benign effects. To our mind, they do more than mislead; they create unrealistic expectations that doom reformist efforts to eventual programmatic failure. The failure-reform cycle breeds not a certain wary skepticism, as seems to be the case with car advertising, but instead dismay and loss of confidence. Programs meant to provide reassurance and security become themselves sources of anxiety—an anxiety that relates both to the stability of personal economic prospects and to the capacity of American government to do a competent job of providing social welfare.

One antidote to the hyperinflation of reform rhetoric is to recognize that fundamental change is virtually never on the political agenda—much less likely to be accomplished. Moreover, rather than being an occasion for further dismay, this situation results from several moderately encouraging aspects of the American welfare state. First, the programs already in place fit fairly well with our political ideology. Junking them in favor of radically different programs would make sense, therefore, only if we experienced some major upheaval in our basic beliefs. And a major shift in beliefs would probably occur only as a result of equally major shifts in our economic, political, or social circumstances. Upheavals such as in the 1930s and, arguably, in the 1960s are rare; for that most of us are thankful. We may praise both the revolutionary spirit and the ultimate outcome of major political, social, or economic rearrangements, but participation in revolutions, or in the economic, political, or social malaise that generates them, is something most people would rather leave to others.

In this book, for example, the most radical change proposed concerns medical care arrangements. That change could be described in stark terms as a shift from a system of private competition in health care provision to a system of public provision or "socialized medicine." Indeed, we have little doubt that, in jockeying for position on the political agenda, demands for "fundamental change" will often attend the reemerging discussion of national health insurance. But this description—"socialized medicine"—vastly overstates the concrete changes necessary to move from our current organization of medical care to one fashioned on the Canadian model. Indeed, it is because we have already moved so far in the direction of health management through bilateral negotiations between insurers and providers that further steps to rationalize and extend the system may become politically feasible.

Second, incrementalism is strongly reinforced by pluralist politics. Programs develop multiple constituencies that must be appeased whenever changes are, in fact, made. Because radical revamping upsets expectations, indeed destroys or transfers economic assets, interest-group politics almost ensures that change will be "balanced." Constituency resistance is, of course, much-lamented by the reform-minded. But stability also has value. Our pluralistic politics means that we are highly unlikely to rationalize the American welfare state on a Swedish Social Democratic model or abolish it in a fit of privatization. We are not even likely to produce the lesser but considerable oscillations that have attended British pensions policy at the hands of alternating Labor and Conservative parliamentary majorities. And from the standpoint of either the well-being of the aged or the general acceptability of programs to the populace at large, avoiding that latter form of instability in programs clearly is an advantage of American political institutions.

A considerable discount must be applied, therefore, to claims of either the need for or the possibility of comprehensive social welfare reform. Most programs that make up the American welfare state have been around for quite a while in one form or another. That form is constantly changing, but almost never radically, whatever ballyhoo attends this or that amendment.

The 1988 reform ("major," "historic," "revolutionary"—choose your adjective) of AFDC provides an excellent example of incrementalism packaged as comprehensive redirection. Presumably the "new consensus" on welfare that resulted in passage of the Family Support Act consisted in a determination (1) that work should be thoroughly integrated with welfare provision and (2) that long-term welfare dependency was an evil demanding serious attention. This consensus was to be implemented by tougher work rules, heavier emphasis on earnings and family responsibility for child support, and parity, if not precedence, for the working poor in the allocation of benefits.

The French, of course, have an expression for such breakthroughs in social engineering—*"plus ça change. . . ."* Since when have Americans *not* worried about the work-welfare trade-off in welfare provision? Since when have we *not* limited provision of aid to those legitimately out of the work force or *not* tried to make payment amounts and conditions reinforce incentives to find work and to leave welfare? Since when have

231

we *not* thought the family and the market the primary defenses against want? Since never. So what actually happened?

In 1988, we began with two sides whose positions had changed little since the 1960s. Conservatives are concerned predominately with budgetary costs and the effects of transfers on the work ethic and traditional family values. Liberals are primarily concerned with adequate benefit levels and the creation of social services and other supportive activities that will increase economic opportunity for the disadvantaged. The state-federal structure is always a complicating factor. But because there are conservative and liberal states, agreement can often be accomplished by leaving certain "new" initiatives to state discretion.

Given this basic structure of contending political forces, certain items are perennially on the agenda: benefit levels, work incentives, work programs, education and training, and, in recent years, pursuit of absent fathers. Each of these issues also carries with it the inevitable state-federal questions of whether program elements will be mandatory or discretionary and how the funding formula for AFDC or any of its subparts will be affected. To the extent there are "new" issues and "new" proposals, they have to do with adjustments across this very stable agenda of policy concerns. The overall conservative or liberal direction of change from every reform effort will generally be quite modest as conservatives and liberals trade their preferred adjustments in one domain for the other's preferred adjustments in another.

The terms of trade can also be specified to some degree in advance. Liberals usually are prepared to accept more stringent work requirements as long as education, training, and job placement are supported more generously. Conservatives generally are prepared to spend additional funds, and even increase benefits, provided that administrative controls are beefed up to detect fraud or error or to pursue support from absent fathers and that state discretion over ultimate payment levels is preserved.

As in any bargaining situation, of course, strange and somewhat surprising things can happen. Whether any new bargain is struck and how it is shaped will depend on a number of unruly factors. Chief among them are the occasion for reform, the current political composition of the Congress (particularly the relevant committee and subcommittee chairs), and the skill (or luck) of the bargainers in shaping the public rhetoric of reform. Welfare reform occasioned by fiscal crises will be different in emphasis from welfare reform attendant on the discovery or rediscovery of poverty. But occasions, personalities, and packaging never generate a permanent victory for either side. The liberals never achieve a federalized and relatively unconditional income support program modeled on the NIT (a program also supported by some libertarians); conservatives never succeed in abolishing welfare in favor of workfare or in returning welfare policy to its pre-1935 jurisdictional home in states and localities.

Moreover, it is often extremely difficult for noncombatants to tell what is going on. Not only is the agenda for reform misrepresented as including, indeed featuring, total revision; the general direction of change is often portrayed in a highly misleading fashion. The Family Support Act of 1988 is a prime example of both tendencies. Not only is this statute really no more than a set of marginal adjustments to existing law; it is also a sheep in wolves' clothing. Portrayed as a move from welfare toward workfare, the Family Support Act is primarily an increase in coverage and benefits.

To be sure, the reform deal this time is contained in a complicated statute. The conference report explaining it runs nearly 140 pages. In that sense it represents a major reform *effort*. But here, as elsewhere, legal complexity is largely a hallmark of continuous refinement and compromise, not of new beginnings. The bill makes adjustments across a wide range of features within the already complex AFDC landscape. To read the conference report, however, is to be impressed, not with radical change, but with continuity. As the report plods forward listing first sections of "Present Law," then the amendments adopted in the House and the Senate, and then the conference agreement, one finds first that "Present Law" is almost never an empty category. This "complete redirection" of welfare policy is really a set of section-by-section amendments. Second, the changes that are made from Present Law could be considered pathbreaking only by those who summoned up the sometimes heroic energies necessary to make even these reforms finally happen.

How does major effort translate into modest reform? The basic story is straightforward. The occasion for the 1988 reforms was in some sense the discovery or rediscovery of the emerging "underclass." Conservatives and liberals, of course, interpreted this discovery as having quite different policy implications. For liberals, the notion that the poor were getting poorer, more desperate, more alienated from the mainstream was but confirmation of their views concerning the likely effects of the neglect of the poverty problem that had been characteristic of the postoil shock, and particularly of the Reagan, period. Funding for a host of supportive services had been slashed. AFDC support levels had been allowed to decline drastically in real terms. There had been federal cutbacks in benefits for the working poor, in Food Stamps, and in Medicaid. It was hardly surprising to the liberals that this neglect was producing an increase in social pathology.

For conservatives the underclass idea resonated with very different preconceptions. Family dissolution, illegitimacy, teenage pregnancy, and work force nonparticipation were (and are) seen as the predictable effects of a welfare system that had progressively decoupled entitlement and responsibility. Conservatives tend to believe Charles Murray's story of Harold and

Phyllis. Indeed, they believed it long before he wrote it. And his view of the steady relaxation of social requirements or conditions on aid matched their own view of the history of welfare in the post-1960s era. A common sense of changed circumstances and new troubles thus provided the occasion for the construction of a reform coalition. The usual possibilities for trade over the standard set of agenda items within AFDC held the coalition together despite its radically differing visions of the causes of the trouble to be addressed.

From the face of the statute, the trades seem to have produced a balanced package. Conservatives got stronger enforcement of child support obligations, increased eligibility of single mothers with small children for mandatory work and training, and mandatory participation in work or training programs by the principal wage earner in all AFDC-UP families. Liberal attempts to put a federal floor under state benefit levels were rejected and states were given additional authority to experiment with novel family support initiatives that integrate and replace existing AFDC, Food Stamp, and other programs, and to limit recipient eligibility for AFDC-UP to six months in each twelve-month period.

From the liberal agenda came the mandating of AFDC-UP in all states, guarantees of child care for participants in mandatory work and training, expanded Medicaid eligibility for families making the transition from welfare to work, and other guarantees or incentives to ensure that work is required only where it involves a financial gain over the receipt of welfare. In addition, substantial new funds are committed to social services and educational efforts in connection with the general thrust toward employment and employability. And, of course, many particular provisions reflect their own internal balance between conservative and liberal preferences.

Why then do we describe the statute as a sheep in wolves' clothing? We do so because the reform was heralded, both in the Congress and out, in conservative terms. Not only was the

"L word" not uttered, the L policies embodied in the act were largely ignored. But even more than that, we think the liberals probably got the better of the bargain because the items chosen from their crucial agenda, the desire to increase benefits, are much easier to implement. There is little reason to doubt that expanded AFDC-UP or Medicaid eligibility will be implemented or that recipients will accept the higher benefits. Most of this is just bookkeeping. And, although we do not want to ignore the difficulties of accomplishing even bookkeeping changes in many state welfare departments, these are the easiest things to alter through bureaucratic routines.

Conservatives, by contrast, will not have succeeded in accomplishing their most basic objective, substituting work for welfare, unless state welfare (and other) departments can make some headway in devising implementable programs for education, training, and placement of those who, by usual workplace standards, are very hard to employ. This is far from easy. Indeed, years of experience in a multitude of jobs programs, within AFDC and outside it, suggest that the "hard core" unemployed are very difficult to train and place. Only the most lavishly funded programs have had demonstrable success. And, of course, lavish funding conflicts with another central conservative preoccupation, cost control.

In the end, the Family Support Act is best understood as a modest expansion of eligibility and benefits targeted primarily on the working poor. It might even be described as merely reinstating, through different means, some of the cuts in benefits for that population that were enacted in the budgetary belt-tightening of the 1981 Omnibus Budget Reconciliation Act. But that would be churlish, and we do not mean to be critical of what the Congress accomplished. Indeed, our objective is quite the opposite. Our fear is that this reform effort, like all others, will be judged a failure instead of a modest success precisely because it will someday—rather soon, we suspect—be discovered not to have completely revamped welfare, eliminated poverty, and consigned the underclass to the dustbin of outmoded ideas. It can avoid that fate only if we will remember that comprehensive reform was not on the agenda. It (almost) never is.

A CODA ON IDEOLOGY

We could continue with a longer list of policy-analytic dos and don'ts. But rules-of-thumb, if multiplied, become a manual suitable mostly for gathering dust. Thumbs are used as rulers, after all, because the complete toolkit is too bulky to carry around. These basic caveats on confusing projections with forecasts, incentives with behaviors, multiple purposes with incoherence, and heroic effort with revolutionary reform are probably sufficient intellectual baggage to ward off the major policy-analytic blunders to which Americans are regularly exposed.

Yet, we cannot close this book without returning to ideology—a topic that appears and reappears throughout the preceding pages. If we had to summarize our message in caveat form, we might put it something like *Rule 5: Ideology Drives Analysis.* But that formulation should not be taken as a blanket criticism. Of course ideology drives analysis. Everyone thinks about public policy on the basis of some set of political preconceptions. How a particular analyst proceeds—what questions are asked, what is identified as relevant and important, how raw data are framed into interpretable patterns, how irreducible uncertainty is managed—will be broadly consistent with the analyst's political ideology. The warning signal in our message on ideology, then, is only to remember that each analyst must have an ideological perspective. Each bit of social welfare policy talk must, therefore, be examined for its ideological perspective. Only in that way can the critical observer begin to understand how such talk is to be interpreted.

In some cases, interpretation through the lens of ideology will reveal conceptual errors. As we saw in chapter 5, for example, social insurance can only be misdescribed if approached from the perspective of individual investment in private insurance. In that case, ideology led to a misunderstanding of program purposes and hence to a failure to appreciate programmatic successes. This privatizing impulse may even make the obvious invisible. To continue with this example, Social Security pensions were credited with the production of national dissavings, although that program's trust funds are, in fact, building up enormous surpluses in a *public* savings account.

In other cases the same ideological perspective—a tendency to see private market institutions and activities as the norm against which a program or policy is to be judged—has less dramatic effects. We believe, for example, that the emphasis on restoring competitiveness in medical care is a bankrupt policy perspective, belied both by foreign experience and by our own modest regulatory successes. But this emphasis on the private market analogy does not fundamentally mischaracterize American health care institutions (the vast majority of which remain privately owned and operated) or American health services (the majority of which are also allocated through market transactions).

In yet other circumstances, attentiveness to ideology merely allows the application of something like an appropriate discount rate. It reminds us that all analysis is interpretative and that the same events or facts will always have multiple meanings or implications for social welfare policy. Thus work requirements in welfare may be viewed by both the Left and the Right as the public assistance system's most important feature. For analysts on the Left, like Frances Fox Piven and Richard Cloward, work requirements epitomize the total social welfare system, a system they believe to be primarily devoted to regulating the poor.[3] For their right-leaning behaviorist colleagues, like Charles Murray, work is also central—because it is the best hope of reforming dependent persons and reintegrating them into the mainstream culture. Meanwhile, contemporary centrist policy analysts like David Ellwood interpret work demands as having a much more modest role in income support.[4] They are necessary to keep faith with the working poor and serve as evidence of a continuing commitment to opportunity and human capital investment in our social welfare arrangements. But required work is not for them a central, defining characteristic of social welfare policy. We would thus do well to attend to several points of view before imagining that we know what has happened, or will happen, as a result of any particular social welfare policy or proposal—or, indeed, as a result of the emergence and growth of the welfare state as a whole.

But, beyond generating yet another prophylactic rule to protect against policy-analytic error, our preceding discussions of ideology point toward a broader conclusion. Social welfare policy is inherently ideological because our social welfare arrangements are ideologically definitional—they say much about who we are as a people and what we believe. It is that aspect of social welfare policy analysis and debate, as much as any other, that gives this arena of public policy its high emotional charge. "What shall we do?" in talking about social welfare provision also implies "Who are we?"—a question that almost no one confronts with complete equanimity.

For Americans, however, thinking about our social welfare arrangements has been more than routinely stressful. Rightist commentators have generally insisted that most of our programs are inconsistent with our dominant individualist and market ideology, not to mention our commitment to limited and decentralized governance. Leftist commentators bemoan our lack of communitarian ideals or our iconoclastic refusal to recognize unavoidable class conflicts that elsewhere buttress and protect welfare state institutions through strong union and labor party organizations. From both perspectives, American social welfare policy arrangements appear fragmented, contradictory, and, ultimately, ideologically incoherent.

239

As we argue most directly in chapter 2, we believe these perspectives misunderstand what American social welfare policy has been about. To be sure, American social welfare programs have combined elements of behaviorist, residualist, social insurance, and even radical populist thinking. But these combinations have been in pursuit of two overarching goals— insurance against common risks and the provision of equal opportunity. Our ideas of what risks are "common" in the sense of "appropriate for universal insurance" and our understanding of how equal opportunity can best be furthered are both constantly evolving. There is much tinkering about the edges of the welfare state as new issues emerge and old problems are seen in the light of new conditions. But social insurance and equal opportunity are our constant social welfare policy commitments, and we return to these guiding ideas time and again as we seek to sort out the appropriate approach to pressing social issues.

Like all such ideas, social insurance and equal opportunity are malleable—but not infinitely so. When viewed within the broader American ideological context, these ideas have a certain integrity and coherence, which also features commitments to individual and family autonomy, market allocation of most goods and services, and limited and decentralized governance. They tell us much about why we have the welfare state arrangements we do and about the probable direction of future developments. These commitments bound the feasible set of policy initiatives. Our political history suggests that they place a generous negative income tax well off the agenda of practical political action. They put the dismantlement of Social Security pensions for the aged or the disabled in the same preposterous proposals.

The insurance-opportunity state is nevertheless hospitable to many new initiatives. Recent recognition of the vastly increased risks of childhood poverty and single parenthood, for example, will surely affect our understanding of what, as a society, we need to be insured against. And, because insurance against being born into a deprived family merges with ideas about equal opportunity through human capital development, additional commitments of resources to combating childhood poverty seem firmly on the agenda of future political action.

As these and other proposals emerge and are debated, they will often be portrayed as pursuing disparate goals—poverty reduction, economic efficiency, family responsibility, and a host of others. Much of this talk may well be true. The social welfare programs that pass through the legislative gauntlet and endure through long periods of implementation, however, are likely to have a common feature: They reflect our enduring commitments to social insurance and equal opportunity, while recognizing that we are also committed to individualism, the market, and limited government.

Notes

Chapter 1

1. The boundaries of "social welfare policy" or of the "welfare state" can be defined in many ways. In Europe, the welfare state is commonly viewed as encompassing not only income-transfer programs but also the production of public goods like education and the regulation of working conditions and employment relations. This book focuses more narrowly on transfer programs alone—both those designed to serve the needs of the population as a whole, like Social Security, and those designed to deliver targeted aid to the needy, like Aid to Families with Dependent Children (AFDC), Medicaid, and Food Stamps (see tables 2.1 and 2.2). We have limited our discussion of American social welfare policy to these programs because they are the focus of the myths, misunderstanding, and misinformation to which this book is a response.

2. Richard E. Cohen, "'Big Government' Emerges as Big Issue in '76 Election Campaign," *National Journal*, 6 March 1976.

3. Robert Walters, "Liberals Disillusioned with Government," *National Journal*, 13 May 1975. This same trend among liberals was described by Bernard Weinraub in *The New York Times* of 28 Dec. 1980 in an article on the emerging strength of neoconservatives, former political liberals whose views on some issues have become more conservative during the past two decades as

a result of their disillusionment with the campus revolts of the 1960s, the rise of the counterculture, the Great Society programs [they] felt were misconceived., etc.

4. Patrick J. Buchanan, for example, described the Great Society as not just a failure but a calamity that converted an improving situation into an unmitigated social disaster. Patrick J. Buchanan, "Welfare Reform Agenda" (*Washington Times,* 25 Jan. 1985).

5. Three important works that attempted to swim against the tidal wave of pessimism are Christopher Jencks, "The Hidden Prosperity of the 1970s," *Public Interest* (Fall 1984): 37–61; John E. Schwarz, *America's Hidden Success: A Reassessment of Public Policy from Kennedy to Reagan,* rev. ed. (New York: Norton, 1987); and Forrest Chisman and Alan Pifer, *Government for the People: The Federal Social Role, What It Is, What It Should Be* (New York: Norton, 1987).

6. Samuel P. Huntington, *American Politics: The Promise of Disharmony* (Cambridge, Mass.: Harvard University Press, 1981), pp. 102–04 and 111–12.

7. Franklin D. Roosevelt, "Annual Message to Congress," *Congressional Record,* vol. 90, part 1, p. 57, col. 1 (January 1944).

8. The same data reveal, for example, that respondents believe Social Security pensions make the elderly more "independent." Fay Lomax Cook, "Congress and the Public: Convergent and Divergent Opinions on Social Security," in *Social Security and the Budget,* ed. Henry Aaron (Lanham, Md.: University Press of America, 1990), pp. 79–107.

9. Median household income continued to grow in the post-1973 period because of continued growth in the median income of nonfamily households (individuals living alone or with other unrelated persons). But because the great bulk of the population (over 85 percent in 1988) lives in families, family income predominates in defining the standard of living of the American population. If more aggregated measures of income change are traced, they show continued growth in the post-1973 period, but at substantially reduced rates. For example, real per capita GNP grew at an average annual rate of 2.2 percent from 1947

to 1973, but at a rate of only 1.4 percent from 1973 to 1987. For a fuller discussion of income trends in the postwar era, see Frank Levy, *Dollars and Dreams: The Changing American Income Distribution* (New York: Russell Sage, 1987).

10. See U.S. Congress, House of Representatives, Committee on Ways and Means, *Background Material and Data on Programs within the Jurisdiction of the Committee on Ways and Means* (Washington, D.C.: GPO, 1989), pp. 983–1018.

11. Charles Murray, *Losing Ground: American Social Policy, 1950–1980* (New York: Basic Books, 1984).

12. Frances Fox Piven and Richard A. Cloward, *Regulating the Poor* (New York: Vintage Books, 1971).

13. James O'Connor, *The Fiscal Crisis of the State* (New York: St. Martin's Press, 1972), especially chap. 6.

14. Martin Feldstein, "Social Security, Induced Retirement, and Aggregate Accumulation," *Journal of Political Economy* 82 (Sept.–Oct. 1974): 905–26.

15. Data from Thomas Edsall, *The New Politics of Inequality* (New York: Norton, 1984), pp. 117–20.

16. Among the books that embody the conservative critique of the welfare state are Martin Anderson, *Welfare: The Political Economy of Welfare Reform in the United States* (Stanford, Calif.: The Hoover Institution, 1978); Roger A. Freeman, *The Growth of American Government: A Morphology of the Welfare State* (Stanford, Calif.: The Hoover Institution, 1975); A. Haeworth Robertson, *The Coming Revolution in Social Security* (Reston, Va.: Reston Publishing Co., 1981); Peter J. Ferrara, *Social Security: The Inherent Contradiction* (Washington, D.C.: The Cato Institute, 1980); George Gilder, *Wealth and Poverty* (New York: Basic Books, 1981); Charles Murray, *Losing Ground;* Peter G. Peterson and Neil Howe, *On Borrowed Time: How the Growth in Entitlement Spending Threatens America's Future* (New York: Simon & Schuster, 1988); and Stuart Butler and Anna Kondratas, *Out of the Poverty Trap: A Conservative Strategy for Welfare Reform* (New York: Free Press, 1987). Lawrence M. Mead's critical treatment of AFDC, *Beyond Entitlement: The Social Obligations of Citizenship*

(New York: The Free Press, 1986), undeniably espouses conservative values, but is far more careful in characterizing America's ideological heritage.

Chapter 2

1. Thomas Malthus, *An Essay on Population* (New York: E. P. Dutton, 1914), vol. 2, p. 170.
2. Malthus, *Essay on Population*, p. 184.
3. Robert T. Kudrle and Theodore R. Marmor, "The Development of the Welfare State in North America," in *The Development of Welfare States in Europe and America*, eds. Peter Flora and Arnold Heidenheimer (New Brunswick, N.J.: Transaction, 1981), pp. 81–121, especially p. 100.
4. A multitude of questions regarding the desirability of redistribution of income and power, however, arise when one considers this conception. Is the welfare state's social insurance designed to bring about adequate subsistence alone, or equity of treatment, or equality of results? Is it to compensate for past social injustice and misfortune or, through the management of large capital funds, to assist future investment? Is it designed to supplement or replace wage income and savings, to redistribute cash, services, or power, and with what balance among them? What links the social insurance advocates, despite their varied answers to these questions, is first the rejection of the behaviorist and the residualist conceptions of welfare and second, hesitancy about how much redistribution of income and power social insurance programs should be expected to accomplish.
5. Theodore R. Marmor, "The North American Welfare State: Social Science and Evaluation," in *Value Judgement and Income Distribution*, eds. Robert A. Solo and Charles W. Anderson (New York: Praeger, 1981), pp. 320–39.
6. Public employees were specifically excluded from coverage under the Social Security Act of 1935. Over the years, they gradually have been brought into the system, but it is still appropriate to regard a portion of the old-age, survivors', and disability pension benefits provided to government employees as functionally equivalent to Social Security payments. Table 2.1

includes an estimate of these Social Security equivalent payments.

7. Submitted to President Roosevelt on 15 January 1935, reprinted in *The 50th Anniversary Edition of the Report of the Committee on Economic Security of 1935 and Other Basic Documents Relating to the Development of the Social Security Act,* eds. Alan Pifer and Forrest Chisman (Washington, D.C.: National Conference on Social Welfare, 1985).

8. *50th Anniversary Edition of the Report of the Committee on Economic Security,* p. 21.

9. Ibid., p. 23.

10. M. Kenneth Bowler, *The Nixon Guaranteed Income Proposal: Substance and Process in Policy Change* (Cambridge, Mass.: Ballinger, 1974); Daniel Patrick Moynihan, *The Politics of a Guaranteed Annual Income: The Nixon Administration and the Family Assistance Plan* (New York: Random House, 1973).

11. *50th Anniversary Edition of the Report of the Committee on Economic Security,* p. 56.

12. See Philip Harvey, *Securing the Right to Employment* (Princeton, N.J.: Princeton University Press, 1989), pp. 99–112.

13. Theodore R. Marmor, *The Politics of Medicare* (Chicago: Aldine, 1973).

14. Fay Lomax Cook, "Congress and the Public: Convergent and Divergent Opinions on Social Security," in *Social Security and the Budget,* ed. Henry J. Aaron (Lanham, Md.: University Press of America, 1990), pp. 79–107.

15. Fay Lomax Cook, Edith J. Barrett, Susan J. Popkin, Ernesto A. Constantino, and Julie E. Kaufman, *Convergent Perspectives on Social Welfare Policy: The Views from the General Public, Members of Congress, and AFDC Recipients* (Evanston, Ill.: Center for Urban Affairs and Policy Research [CUAPR] Research Reports, 1988), pp. 3–59 and 3–60.

16. If one merely reviewed the empirical work of persons associated with the Wisconsin Institute for Research on Poverty, for example, much of what passes for knowledge or fact in public debates concerning "poverty" policies would rapidly be called into question. See, for example, Sheldon Danziger and

Daniel Weinberg, eds., *Fighting Poverty: What Works and What Doesn't* (Cambridge, Mass.: Harvard University Press, 1987); Robert Havemann, ed., *A Decade of Federal Anti-Poverty Programs: Achievements, Failures, and Lessons* (New York: Academic Press, 1977); Robert Plotnick and Felicity Skidmore, *Progress Against Poverty: A Review of the 1964–74 Decade* (New York: Academic Press, 1975); and David T. Ellwood, *Poor Support: Poverty in the American Family* (New York: Basic Books, 1988).

Chapter 3

1. Claus Offe, *Contradictions of the Welfare State* (Cambridge, Mass.: MIT Press, 1984), p. 153.
2. Lester Thurow, *The Zero-Sum Society* (New York: Basic Books, 1980), p. 12.
3. See Daniel Hamermesh, *Jobless Pay and the Economy* (Baltimore, Md.: Johns Hopkins University Press, 1977), chap. 3.
4. Henry J. Aaron and Lawrence W. Thompson, "Social Security and the Economists," in *Social Security After 50: Successes & Failures,* ed. Edward D. Berkowitz (Westport, Conn.: Greenwood Press, 1987), p. 91.
5. Subrata N. Chakravarty with Kathering Weisman, "Consuming Our Children," *Forbes Magazine,* reprinted in *The Generational Journal* (1989): 52–58.
6. *Background Material and Data on Programs within the Jurisdiction of the Committee on Ways and Means,* (Washington, D.C.: GPO, 1989) p. 89, table 13.
7. See Richard Rose and Guy Peters, *Can Government Go Bankrupt?* (New York: Basic Books, 1978).
8. The 50 percent figure includes a number of programs that are largely beyond the scope of this book (such as education expenditures, veterans' programs, medical research, medical facilities construction, and Defense Department medical expenditures). If only Old-Age, Survivors', Disability, Health Insurance (OASDHI), Unemployment Insurance (UI), workers' compensation, and all means-tested programs (except for education aid) are included, the total bill came to 35 percent of

federal expenditures in 1986 and 31 percent of all government expenditures.

9. Rudolf Klein and Michael O'Higgins, "Defusing the Crisis of the Welfare State: A New Interpretation," in *Social Security: Beyond the Rhetoric of Crisis,* eds. Theodore R. Marmor and Jerry L. Mashaw (Princeton, N.J.: Princeton University Press, 1988), pp. 203–25.

Chapter 4

1. Family Support Act of 1988, Public Law No. 100–485, 102 Stat. 2343 (1988).

2. The social welfare category used here is a somewhat broader one than we have been using to define the American welfare state. In addition to the expenditures detailed in tables 2.1 and 2.2, the figures in table 4.1 include outlays for federal civil service and military pensions not included in table 2.1, Defense Department medical expenditures, educational assistance to local school systems, support for medical research, and subsidies for the construction of health care facilities. In 1986, when federal spending for the programs included in tables 2.1 and 2.2 totaled $415.6 billion, federal social welfare spending totaled $472.4 billion.

3. Nor, as we have seen, do *federal* outlays constitute all welfare state expenditures. Tables 2.1 and 2.2 show that state and local spending added $93.1 billion to the $415.6 billion spent by the federal government on transfer programs in 1986. When the welfare state is defined more broadly in the manner of table 4.1, state and local spending takes on much greater importance. In 1986, state and local governments spent $163.5 billion on education, $25 billion on public employee pensions, and $24.4 billion on health and medical programs other than Medicaid, and on General Assistance. When spending on these and other similar items is counted, social welfare expenditures by state and local governments totaled $298.2 billion that year, about 39 percent of the combined total for such expenditures by all levels of government.

4. This common view is illustrated in a story by Daniel Wright, a

public relations expert, in "Workfare: A Fine Idea in Need of Work," *Fortune*, 24 Oct. 1988, pp. 213–15, where he writes that the "costs of *welfare* in our economy are becoming intolerable" (our emphasis).

5. See Michael R. Sosin, "Legal Rights and Welfare Change, 1960–1980," in *Fighting Poverty: What Works and What Doesn't*, eds. S. H. Danziger and D. H. Weinberg (Cambridge, Mass.: Harvard University Press, 1986), and James T. Paterson, *America's Struggle Against Poverty, 1900–1980* (Cambridge, Mass.: Harvard University Press, 1981), p. 179.

6. Eugene Durman, "Have the Poor Been Regulated? Toward a Multivariate Theory of Welfare Growth," *Social Service Review* 47 (1973): 339–59.

7. For more about this controversial subject, see Theodore R. Marmor, "The Politics of Welfare Reform," *New Generation* 52 (Winter 1970): 1; Bowler, *Nixon Guaranteed Income Proposal;* Daniel Patrick Moynihan, *The Politics of a Guaranteed Annual Income;* and Nicholas Lemann, "The Unfinished War," *The Atlantic Monthly*, Dec. 1988, pp. 37–56 and Jan. 1989, pp. 53–68. Arguments against guaranteed income plans did not preclude, in principle, the federalization of welfare programs, which by itself would be a substantial improvement. See figure 4.2.

8. Library of Congress, Congressional Research Service, *Cash and Noncash Benefits for Persons with Limited Income: Eligibility Rules, Recipient and Expenditure Data, FY 1986–88* (24 Oct. 1989), p. 9, table 4.

9. The methodology used to calculate the poverty threshold is primitive and there is good reason to believe that it results in a poverty threshold that is too low. Poverty thresholds are calculated by multiplying a basic food budget for families of various sizes by a factor of three. There are several problems with this rough and ready technique. First, the food budget on which it is based is a meager one that does not satisfy all nutritional requirements and is not deemed adequate for long-term use. The USDA originally described it as "designed for temporary or emergency use when funds are low." (U.S. Department of Agriculture, *Family Economics Review*, Oct. 1964, p. 12.)

Second, the "three times the food budget" methodology is also problematic. The factor of three was selected because a 1955 USDA survey of all nonfarm families of four found that they spent an average of 33 percent of their income on food. However, a 1961 USDA survey of *urban* families found that only 19.3 percent of their total personal income, 21.9 percent of their disposable income, and 24.3 percent of their total expenditures went for food. (See ibid., p. 5.) The question thus arises, why wasn't a more adequate food plan used to calculate the poverty threshold, or a factor of 4 to 5 used to calculate the threshold instead of the factor of 3? Either of these methodologies would have resulted in a poverty rate roughly twice as high as the one reported by the government, and that simple statistic may be the answer. To fight a war against poverty on behalf of 20 percent of the population seemed reasonable. To do so on behalf of 40 percent of the population might not have been politically palatable.

The creation of a number of in-kind support programs since 1964 (Food Stamps, energy assistance, Medicaid, etc.) may have partially offset these criticisms. Indeed, welfare state critics sometimes claim that the poverty line is now too high because it ignores the possible receipt of in-kind support. But the United States is virtually alone in using an absolute definition of poverty. Socially and psychologically, poverty is a relative concept. The poverty line as percentage of average income fell sharply in the 1960s. If one makes this adjustment to the baseline, then the United States record of poverty reduction is less impressive.

10. *Background Material and Data on Programs within the Jurisdiction of the Committee on Ways and Means* (Washington, D.C.: GPO, 1989), pp. 962–63, table 16.
11. Ibid.
12. Ibid.; *U.S. Statistical Abstract* (1989), tables 570, 571, and 594.
13. *Statistical Abstract* (1989), table 570.
14. Isabel V. Sawhill, "Poverty in the U.S.: Why Is It So Persistent," *Journal of Economic Literature* 26 (Sept. 1988): 1100.
15. Charles Murray, *Losing Ground: American Social Policy, 1950–1980* (New York: Basic Books, 1984).

16. Sara McLanahan et al., "Losing Ground: A Critique," *IRP Special Report* No. 38, Aug. 1985; "Are We Losing Ground?" *Focus* 8 (Fall and Winter 1985): 1–12; and Christopher Jencks, "How Poor Are the Poor?" *New York Review of Books,* 9 May 1985.

17. *Background Material and Data,* p. 539, table 9.

18. In the early 1980s, David Ellwood and Mary Jo Bane, prompted by the sorts of criticisms Murray voiced, undertook a major study of AFDC benefits and recipients. Their findings provide the basis for many of the conclusions we present here. David T. Ellwood and Mary Jo Bane, "The Impact of AFDC on Family Structure and Living Arrangements," Report Prepared for U.S. Department of Health and Human Services under Grant No. 92A–82, Harvard University, March 1984. See the discussion of numerous other studies in William Julius Wilson and Kathryn M. Neckerman, "Poverty and Family Structure: The Widening Gap between Evidence and Public Policy Issues," in Danziger and Weinberg, *Fighting Poverty,* pp. 248–51.

19. Ellwood and Bane, "The Impact of AFDC." Moreover, in the period in which the percent of children in single parent families went up the most, 1972 to 1980, the percent of children in AFDC families remained constant, a peculiar result if AFDC payments were the causative factor in family formation or disolution. See David T. Ellwood and Lawrence H. Summers, "Poverty in America: Is Welfare the Answer or the Problem?" in Danziger and Weinberg, *Fighting Poverty,* pp. 93–94.

20. Jencks, "How Poor Are the Poor?" pp. 41, 45.

21. Ellwood and Bane, "The Impact of AFDC."

22. Sawhill, "Poverty in the U.S.," p. 1090.

23. Ibid., pp. 1086–88.

24. For a brief review of the literature analyzing this trend, see ibid., pp. 1090–92. For data on trends in pretransfer income inequality from 1979 to 1987, see *Background Material and Data,* pp. 1019–31.

25. E. R. Ricketts and I. Sawhill, "Defining and Measuring the Underclass," *Journal of Policy Analysis and Management* 7

(1988): 316–25. See also "New Studies Zeroing In on the Poorest of the Poor," *New York Times,* 20 Dec. 1987, p. 26, col. 1.
26. Daniel Patrick Moynihan, "Half the Nation's Children: Born Without a Fair Chance," *The New York Times,* 25 Sept. 1988, Sec. 4, p. 25, col. 1
27. Ibid.
28. *Background Material and Data,* p. 594, and table 20, p. 559.
29. Exemptions from participation will be available to persons who are (1) ill, incapacitated, or of advanced age; (2) needed at home because of the illness or incapacity of another member of the household; (3) caring for a young child (under age 3, or a younger age selected by the state, but not under age 1); (4) already working 30 or more hours a week; (5) under age 16 or attending an elementary, secondary, or vocational school full-time; (6) in at least their second trimester of pregnancy; or (7) residing in an area where no training and placement program is available. See *Background Material and Data,* p. 593.
30. For data on the trend in the United States, see U.S. Congress, House of Representatives, Select Committee on Children, Youth, and Families, *U.S. Children and Their Families: Current Conditions and Recent Trends, 1989,* 101st Cong., 1st Sess., Sept. 1989, pp. 14–15.

Chapter 5

1. Board of Trustees of the Federal Old-Age and Survivors Insurance and Disability Insurance Trust Funds, *1988 Annual Report,* table 23, p. 64. The yearly surplus in 1987 was nearly $22 billion and is projected to be over $40 billion in 1988.
2. *The New York Times,* editorial, 11 April 1988, p. A18.
3. Fay Cook, "Congress and the Public."
4. Peter G. Peterson, "The Morning After," *The Atlantic Monthly,* Oct. 1987, pp. 43–69. These arguments are elaborated in his later book with Neil Howe, *On Borrowed Time: How the Growth in Entitlement Spending Threatens America's Future* (San Francisco, Calif.: ICS Press, 1988).
5. Peterson, "The Morning After," p. 43.
6. Peterson and Howe, *On Borrowed Time.* By "entitlements"

Peterson and Howe mean benefit programs for which expenditure levels depend on the number of eligible persons who apply rather than on fixed appropriations. This legal/budgetary usage of the term ought not to be confused with the more commonly understood meaning of entitlement as a benefit that is earned by virtue of financial contributions (Social Security) or special sacrifices (veterans' programs).

7. Peterson, "The Morning After," pp. 60–61.
8. Henry J. Aaron and Robert D. Reischauer, "Bite the Deficit, Not Social Security," *Washington Post,* 16 Dec. 1987.
9. Peterson, "The Morning After," p. 44.
10. Martin Feldstein, "Social Security, Induced Retirement, and Aggregate Accumulation," *Journal of Political Economy* 82 (Sept.-Oct. 1974) 905–26.
11. James Tobin, "The Future of Social Security: One Economist's Assessment," in *Social Security: Beyond the Rhetoric of Crisis,* eds. Theodore R. Marmor and Jerry L. Mashaw (Princeton, N.J.: Princeton University Press, 1988), p. 55.
12. Ibid.
13. Ibid.
14. Ibid.
15. David Wessel, "Social Security: Myths and Moynihan," *The Wall Street Journal,* 15 Jan. 1990, p. 1, col. 5.
16. Peterson and Howe, *On Borrowed Time,* p. 11.
17. These "intermediate" assumptions are actually quite conservative. GNP is projected to grow at an average annual rate of about 2.5 percent during the 1990s, about 2.2 percent during the first decade of the next century, and about 1.9 percent thereafter. This assumes poorer economic performance over the next seventy-five years than we have experienced since 1973. The inflation and unemployment projections are for price increases of about 4 percent per year and an average unemployment rate of about 6 percent with an average annual increase in real wages of about 1.4 percent. See *Background Material and Data on Programs within the Jurisdiction of the Committee on Ways and Means* (Washington, D.C.: GPO, 1989), table 12, pp. 87–88.

18. Peterson and Howe, *On Borrowed Time,* p. 43.
19. Lawrence H. Thompson, "The Financing Debate: A Score-card," based on a speech to the Second Annual Conference of the National Academy of Social Insurance, published in *Perspectives* (National Academy of Social Insurance: Washington, D.C., 1990).
20. GAO, *The Trust Fund Accumulation, The Economy and the Federal Budget* (Jan. 1989): 43.
21. Robert J. Samuelson, "The Elderly Aren't Needy," *Newsweek,* 21 March 1988.
22. "When Social Security's Anti-Social," *The New York Times,* 8 Feb. 1987.
23. Aaron and Reischauer, "Bite the Deficit."
24. James Dale Davidson, "Social Security Rip-Off," *The New Republic,* 11 Nov. 1985, pp. 12–13.
25. "When Social Security's Anti-Social."
26. Ibid.
27. Samuelson, "The Elderly Aren't Needy."
28. "When Social Security's Anti-Social."
29. Ferrara's books and edited volumes on Social Security include: *Social Security: The Inherent Contradiction* (Washington, D.C.: The Cato Institute, 1980); *Social Security: Averting the Crisis* (Washington, D.C.: The Cato Institute, 1982); and *Social Security: Prospects for Real Reform* (Washington, D.C.: The Cato Institute, 1985).
30. Aaron and Reischauer, "Bite the Deficit."
31. Tobin, "Future of Social Security," p. 54.
32. *Background Material and Data,* p. 26, table 13.
33. Aaron and Reischauer, "Bite the Deficit."
34. Merton Bernstein and Joan Broadshaug Bernstein, *Social Security: The System That Works* (New York: Basic Books, 1988), p. 17.
35. See, for example, Martha Derthick, *Policymaking for Social Security* (Washington, D.C.: The Brookings Institution, 1978), and W. Andrew Achenbaum, *Social Security Visions and Revisions* (New York: Cambridge University Press, 1986).

Chapter 6

1. Data for 1966 from *Health, United States, 1986* (Washington, D.C.: GPO, 1986), table 89, p. 183. Data for 1986 and 1987 from *Medical Benefits, The Medical-Economic Digest,* 15 Feb. 1987 and 1988. Figures were deflated using the Consumer Price Index for "all items." If the medical care price index is used instead, the increase in total health care spending was still in excess of 100 percent between 1966 and 1986.

2. *Medical Benefits,* 15 February 1988, p. 3.

3. R. G. Evans et al., "Controlling Health Expenditures: The Canadian Reality," *New England Journal of Medicine* 320 (2 March 1989): 571–77.

4. "National Health Expenditures, 1986–2000," *Health Care Financing Review* 8 (Summer 1987): 24, table 12.

5. For data on relative price index changes, see *Statistical Abstract of the United States: 1988,* table 738, p. 450.

6. *Health, United States, 1986,* tables 12 and 13, pp. 84 and 85.

7. See Diana B. Dutton, *Worse Than the Disease: Pitfalls of Medical Progress* (New York: Cambridge University Press, 1988).

8. See Ivan Illich, *Medical Nemesis: The Expropriation of Health* (New York: Pantheon, 1976). See also Victor Fuchs, *Who Shall Live: Health, Economics, and Social Choice* (New York: Basic Books, 1974) for the argument that what we spend on medical care has less effect on our health than do our heredity, environment, and style of living.

9. Edward Kennedy, *In Critical Condition: The Crisis in America's Health Care* (New York: Simon & Schuster, 1972).

10. Theodore R. Marmor, "Rethinking National Health Insurance," *The Public Interest* 46 (1977): 73–93.

11. Even the exceptional state programs that address access have this character. In 1988, for example, Massachusetts passed a law mandating businesses of a certain size to provide health insurance to their employees and established an insurance pool financed by employer contributions for the unemployed and others who fall outside this plan. Rather than addressing a

social need through public provision, that state has extruded it onto private industry.

12. Paul Starr, *The Social Transformation of American Medicine* (New York: Basic Books, 1982).

13. See Theodore R. Marmor, Mark Schlesinger, and Richard Smithey, "A New Look at Nonprofits: Health Care Policy in a Competitive Age," *Yale Journal on Regulation* 3 (Spring 1986): 313, and Bradford H. Gray, *The New Health Care for Profit: Doctors and Hospitals in a Competitive Environment* (Washington, D.C.: National Academy Press, 1983).

14. In the early 1970s, for instance, Martin Feldstein proposed a version of national health insurance for catastrophic medical costs, which required a deductible set at 10 percent of a family's taxable income. Although widely discussed in the technical literature, this proposed answer to the moral hazard problem failed politically.

15. See Morris L. Barer, Robert G. Evans, and Roberta J. Labelle, "Fee Controls as Cost Control: Tales from the Frozen North," *The Milbank Quarterly* 66 (1988): 1–64.

16. See, for example, Milt Freudenheim, "Health Insurers' Changing Roles," *The New York Times,* 16 Jan. 1990, p. D2, col. 1.

17. Marc Lalonde, *A New Perspective on the Health of Canadians* (Ottawa: Information Canada, 1974).

18. Ivan Illich, *Medical Nemesis: The Expropriation of Health Care* (New York: Pantheon, 1976); Paul Starr and Theodore Marmor, "The United States: A Social Forecast," in *The End of an Illusion: The Future of Health Policy in Western Industrialized Nations,* eds. Jean de Kervasdoué, John R. Kimberly, and Victor G. Rodwin (Berkeley: University of California Press, 1984), p. 236.

19. In one year, from 1970 to 1971, for example, the *Congressional Record* noted 50 references to national health insurance; between 1981 and 1986 there were none. Howard M. Leichter, *Free to Be Foolish? Politics and Changing Lifestyles in Britain and the United States* (Princeton University Press, in press).

20. Louise Russell, *Is Prevention Better Than Cure?* (Washington, D.C.: The Brookings Institution, 1986).

21. Leichter, *Free to Be Foolish?*
22. See Robert Y. Shapiro and John T. Young, "The Polls: Medical Care in the United States," *Public Opinion Quarterly* 50 (1986): 418–28, and Dennis Hevesi, "Polls Show Discontent with Health Care," *The New York Times,* 15 Feb. 1989, p. A16, col. 1.
23. Robert G. Evans, "Improving Access to Affordable Health Care: Lessons from Canada," 1989–90 Richard & Hinda Rosenthal Lecture, Institute of Medicine, April 10, 1989, ms. p. 14.
24. Ibid., p. 573.
25. Administrative costs have become, as of 1990, a regular part of the debate about American medical care. See Evans et al., "Controlling Health Expenditures—The Canadian Reality," pp. 571–77, and D. U. Himmelstein and S. Woolhandler, "Cost without Benefit: Administrative Waste in U.S. Health Care," *New England Journal of Medicine* 314 (1986): 441–45. For a more journalistic presentation of the problem, see M. Freudenheim, "Job Growth in Health Care Soars," *The New York Times,* 5 March 1990, p. D1.
26. For more on the history of the Canadian system, see Malcolm G. Taylor, *Health Insurance and Canadian Public Policy: The Seven Decisions That Created the Canadian Health Insurance System* (Montreal: McGill-Queen's University Press, 1978), and Robert G. Evans and Greg L. Stoddart, eds., *Medicare at Maturity: Achievements, Lessons & Challenges* (Calgary, Alberta: The University of Canada Press, 1986). For the developments of the 1970s and 1980s, see Robert G. Evans, *Strained Mercy: The Economics of Canadian Health Care* (Toronto, Ont.: Butterworths, 1984). And for a critical perspective that does not embrace U.S. patterns, see Michael Rachlis and Carol Kushner, *Second Opinion: What's Wrong with Canada's Health-Care System and How to Fix It* (Toronto, Ont.: Collins Publishers, 1989).
27. Robert G. Evans, "Common Misperceptions about the Canadian Health Care System," draft article. For an extended presentation of these arguments, see Robert G. Evans, "Tension, Compression, and Shear: Directions, Stresses, and Outcomes of

Health Care Cost Control," *Journal of Health Policy, Politics and Law*, 1990, Vol. 15, No. 1, 101-128.

This section has reiterated many of the arguments, and used some of the language, of earlier papers and articles on Canadian national health insurance by Robert Evans, Morris Barer, and their colleagues at the University of British Columbia's health policy research unit. The longstanding collaboration between Marmor and this group (1975 to present) means that it is almost impossible to sort out who said what first.

28. Milt Freudenheim, "Insurers Seek Help for Uninsured," *The New York Times*, 11 Jan. 1990, p. D1, col. 1.

Chapter 7

1. Making the incentives-equal-behaviors mistake, we hasten to add, is not the exclusive province of the conservative or economically oriented analysts who oppose social welfare programs. Leftist commentators can create their own mythologies on the basis of the same false equation: for example, that welfare levels are a straightforward function of the ruling classes' joint desire to maintain low wage levels while avoiding violent social unrest. Compare Francis Fox Piven and Richard A. Cloward, *Regulating the Poor: The Functions of Public Welfare* (New York: Pantheon, 1971) with Eugene Durman, "Have the Poor Been Regulated? Toward a Multivariate Understanding of Welfare Growth," *Social Service Review* 47 (1973): 339–59.

2. Edward D. Berkowitz, *Disabled Policy: America's Programs for the Handicapped* (New York: Cambridge University Press, 1987), p. 4.

3. See Piven and Cloward, *Regulating the Poor*.

4. See David T. Ellwood, *Poor Support: Poverty in the American Family* (New York: Basic Books, 1988).

Index

INDEX

Family: autonomy, 240; cash assistance, 86; characteristics of, 38; as contributor to poverty, 24–25; dissolution of, 234; "dual family system", 118; food budget, 249–50n9; income inequality, 8–12; life cycle, 115; median family income, 9, 70, 71, 217, 226, 243–44n9; size of, 38; solidarity, view of, 4–5; as threat to economic security, 27; weakening of ties, 6. *See also* Aid to Families with Dependent Children (AFDC); Family Support Act of 1988; Single parent family

Family Support Act of 1988, 83, 90, 116, 236; creation of, 231; illegitimacy and poverty, 119–21, 123; reform, 233; shifts in emphasis, 126; training and placement, 122. *See also* JOBS; AFDC

Farmworkers: health care centers for, 91

FDA. *See* Food and Drug Administration

Federal Insurance Contributions Act (FICA), 27; deductions, 132–33, 143; equity issues, 173; impact of tax, 172; projection of taxes, 152–53; public opinion, 160; rate of tax, 147; reduction of taxes, 147, 166; tax revenue, 171

Federal Reserve Board, 61

Feldstein, Martin, 15, 142–43, 256n14

Female-headed households. *See* Single-parent families

Ferrara, Peter, 161–65

Fertility rates, 73–74; forecasting, 217

FICA. *See* Federal Insurance Contributions Act (FICA)

The Fiscal Crisis of the State (O'Connor), 14

Food and Drug Administration, 189

Food Stamp Plan, 22, 40, 91; attitudes towards, survey of, 47–49; cuts in funding, 234; expenditures, 92;

growth of program, 124; replacement of program, 235; single-parent families, 116; unaffordability, 70

Ford, Gerald: state activism, retreat from, 31

Forecasting: projections vs., 216–19; Social Security, 72, 134–35, 137–41, 147–54; social welfare policy, 216–19

Foster grandparents program, 91

France: labor market, 121; medical care expenditures, 175–76, 199–200

Freedom: individual, 6–7, 12

Friedman, Milton, 16

General Accounting Office, 154

General Assistance programs, 38

Gilder, George, 12

GNP. *See* Gross National Product (GNP)

Government employees: fringe benefits, 27; old-age pensions, 33

Gramm, Phil, 145

Great Britain: health insurance, 192; labor market, 121; medical care expenditures, 176, 199–200; origins of welfare state, 53; "poor law" tradition, 25; social welfare policy, 231

"Great Society" programs, 1, 3, 12, 41, 87–88, 91, 182, 243n3–4

Gross National Product (GNP), 61, 64; commitment to social welfare, 72; contributions to social welfare, 86, 87; growth, 58–59, 77, 80, 94, 243–44n9, 253n17; medical care expenses, 175, 179, 197, 199; savings and, 141, 142

Guaranteed Student Loans. *See* Stafford Loans

Handicapped. *See* Disabled persons

Head Start, 42, 91

INDEX

Preventive health care, 193–94
Productivity, effect of welfare state on 54, 58–69, 74, 141–47
Professional Standards Review Organizations, 183
Projection versus forecasting, 216–19
Protest movements, 14
Public debate on social welfare policy, 1–21, 216, 246–47n16
Public employees: Social Security, 245–46n6. *See also* Government employees
Public health, 177, 191. *See also* Medical care
Public opinion: Aid to Families with Dependent Children (AFDC), 82; children, assistance to, 48; disabled persons, assistance to, 48; economists, 219; education programs, 48; elderly, assistance to, 48; Federal Insurance Contributions Act, 160; Kennedy, John F., 4; medical care, 48; Northwestern University, survey of attitudes, 47–49, 103; Reagan, Ronald W., 4; Social Security, 132–36, 177; social welfare policy, 1–21, 103, 216

Race relations, 43, 182
Railroad Retirement program, 33, 149
Rational discourse, need for, 49–52
Reagan, Ronald W.: "boom" years, 60; budget deficit, 183; competition in medicine, 185; Council of Economic Advisers, 15; criticism of social welfare, 12; cuts in funding, 234; fiscal policies, 154; public opinion, 4; Social Security commitment, 75, 138, 139; state activism, retreat from, 31; tax policy, 166; "war on Washington", 1–2
Recession, 8, 58–60, 61

Redistribution of income, 28, 56, 157, 245n4
Reforms in social welfare policy, 3–4, 83, 87, 89, 115, 214, 228–37; Aid to Families with Dependent Children (AFDC), 231; medical care, 183, 209, 210, 229, 230; rhetoric, political, 229–30; Social Security, 128, 131
Refugees: social services for, 91–92
Regulating the Poor (Piven and Cloward), 14
Reischauer, Robert, 140–41, 155–56
Report of the Committee on Economic Security, 33–35, 39–40, 81
Residualist view of social welfare policy, 25–26, 157–58
Responsibility: individual, 6
Retirement rate, 71–72
Roosevelt, Franklin D.: Committee on Economic Security, 33; "State of the Union Message," 1944, 7
Rudman, Warren B., 145
Rural areas: housing repair loans, 91; poverty, 42

Safety laws, 193
Samuelson, Robert, 155, 158–59
Savings rates, 245n4; national savings, 141–44; private savings, 144; Social Security and, 141–44, 221; social welfare expenditures and, 67–69
School Lunch Program, 91
Seamen's hospitals: medical care, 178
Self-help, 43
Single-parent families, 41, 106, 116, 120, 240–41, 251n19
Smoking restrictions, 193
Social insurance programs, 240, 245n4; core commitment, 31–34; expansion of, 104; expenditures, table of, 32; poverty reduction and, 99–100, 102; savings rates, 67; taxa-